INTELLIGENT COI

ALZHEIMER'S I

S. NAGANANDHINI

TABLE OF CONTENTS

CHAPTER NO	TITLE	PAGE NO

LIST OF ALGORITHMS

LIST OF ABBREVIATIONS

MRI	Magnetic Resonance Imaging
fMRI	Function Magnetic Resonance Imaging
sMRI	Structural Magnetic Resonance Imaging
CT	Computed Tomography
PET	Positron Emission Tomography
DIP	Digital Image Processing
NIH-NIA	National Institutes of Health–National Institute on Aging
IBSR	Internet Brain Segmentation Repository
MIRIAD	Minimal Interval Resonance Imaging in Alzheimer Disease
OASIS	Open Access Series of Imaging Studies
ADNI	Alzheimer's Disease Neuroimaging Initiative
AD	Alzheimer's Disease
HC	Healthy Control
VMAD	Very Mild Alzheimer's Disease
WM	White Matter
GM	Gray Matter
CSF	Cerebrospinal Fluid
MSA-C	Multiple System Atrophy- Cerebellum
CAD	Computer-Aided Detection
CDR	Clinical Dementia Ratio
MMSE	Mini-Mental State Examination
ACM	Active Contour Method
EM	Expectation Maximization
NLM	Non-Local Median Filter
TP	True Positive
TN	True Negative
FP	False Positive
FN	False Negative
MCI	Mild Cognitive Impairment

M	Moderate
S	Severe
FAR	False acceptance rate
FRR	False rejection rate
AHE	Adaptive histogram equalization
FCLMS	Fuzzy clustering with level set
SVM	Support vector machine
P	Precision
R	Recall
F	F1-Score
RNLM	Recursive Non-Local Median Filter
RFC	Random Forest Classifier
MLP	Multi-Layer Perception
AdaBoost	Adaptive Boosting Classifier
DTC	Decision Tree Classifier
MDTC	Modified Decision Tree Classifier
GBC	Gradient Boosting Classifier
ETC	Extra Tree Classifier
XGB	Extreme Gradient Boosting
GPC	Gaussian Processing Classifier
K-NN	K-Nearest-Neighbours
CNN	Convolutional Neural Network
R-NN	Recurrent Neural Network
TL	Transfer Learning
KM	K-Means Clustering
DNN	Deep Neural Network
MNLR	Multinomial Logistic Regression
LR	Logistic Regression
CM	Confusion Matrix
CR	Classification Report
MAE	Mean Absolute Error

MSE	Mean Square Error
CPP	Combined Patch Pixel
DSI	Dice Similarity Index
CLAHE	Contrast Limited Adaptive Histogram Equalization
FP-ANN	Feed Forward Back-Propagation Artificial Neural Network
ANN	Artificial Neural Network
DWT	Discrete Wavelet Transform
SOM	Self-Organizing Map
PCA	Principal Component Analysis
RBM	Restricted Boltzmann Machine
ANFIS	Adaptive Neuro-Fuzzy Inference System
RELM	Regularized Extreme Learning Machine
CMA	Centre for Morphometry Analysis
IVM	Import Vector Machine
AAL	Automatic Anatomical Labelling
GIS	Geographical Information Systems
RCNN	Recurrent Convolutional Neural Network
RoI	Regions of Interest
KMEM	K-Means and Expectation Maximization Clustering
TMOS	Thresholded Morphological Operation Based Segmentation
MAP	Maximum A Posterior
BLR	Binary Logistic Regression
NB	Naïve Bayes
GB	Gaussian Bayes
eTIV	Estimated Total Intracranial Volume
nWBV	Normalized Whole-brain Volume
PCS	Post-Concussion Syndrome
EC	Ensemble Classifier
MRF	Modified Random Forest Classifier
MGBC	Modified Gradient Boosting Classifier

LIST OF SYMBOLS

SYMBOLS	DESCRIPTION
$f(x, y)$	Two-dimensional Function
(x, y)	Coordinate
$R_I(I - p)$	Morphological Reconstruction and Dilations on the Image I with respect to $(I - p)$
(T_1, T_2)	MRI Brain Thresholding
I	MRI Brain Image
I_F	Filtered Image
σ_j^2	Covariance
f_{n+1}	distribution over the latent variable
I_{RE}	Brain Region Extracted Image

CHAPTER 1

INTRODUCTION

A digital image is a visual representation of an object or scene. It is composed of essential elements called a pixel, characterized as f (x,y), where f denotes the amplitude and (x,y) is its unique spatial coordinates. The process of converting an analog image into a digital image is called Image Digitization that involves sampling and quantization. Sampling determines a digital image's spatial coordinates, whereas quantization assigns integer values for the sampled amplitude of the image at the sampled spatial coordinates [*Milan Sonka et al., 2008]*.

1.1 MEDICAL IMAGING

Medical image is a type of digital image processing that has widened its boundaries over the decades. It is a primary source for the visual representation of a human system's internal organs for clinical interpretation and intervention. The growth and developments in this field have triggered the development of novel algorithms for data/ image processing.

The medical imaging modalities are medical imaging and processing, Structural Magnetic Resonance Imaging (sMRI), Functional Magnetic Resonance Imaging (fMRI), Digital Mammogram, Ultra Sound (US), Positron Emission Tomography (PET), Electrocardiogram (ECG), and Computer Tomography (CT) that have promoted research in many allied fields including Geographical Information Systems (GIS), Forensic Science, Business Data Analytics and Astronomy. Digital Image is mathematically represented as a two-dimensional function, f(x, y) where x and y are the spatial coordinates, and the amplitude f at any given pair of coordinates (x, y) is called intensity. Digital Image Processing (DIP) is the subject area that deals with processing/ manipulating a digital image by a digital computer to obtain useful and necessary information from it. The different elements of a DIP system include image acquisition, image storage, and image processing [*Richard E. Woods, 2009]*.

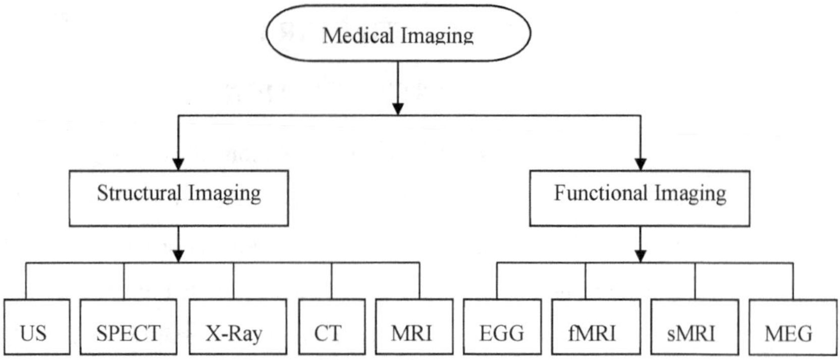

Fig. 1.1 Types of Neuroimaging

1.2 MEDICAL IMAGE PROCESSING

Medical image processing is an offshoot of DIP, which involves using technology to process the human body's medical images. Medical imaging is also referred to as diagnostic imaging. Medical imaging aims to visualize the human body's inner parts, which is required to identify internal abnormalities such as broken bones, tumors, and leaking blood vessels. In medical imaging, segmentation aims to study anatomical structure, demarcate and distinguish a region and help in therapeutic planning and treatment.

Recent medical image diagnosis encompasses the advancement of the latest technology for acquiring the medical images by different modalities used for diagnosis, treatment, and research. Medical image processing covers a broad array of operations categorized as low-level, mid-level, and high-level image processing based on computation complexity. Medical image segmentation contributes to analyzing human anatomy and diagnosing the disorders, using automated or semi-automated computational systems. The foremost objective of medical image segmentation is to extract the regions to study the intrinsic anatomical structure and estimate the severity of abnormalities that help in deciding the means and methods of treatment. These aspects motivate researchers to develop competent computing techniques for pre-processing, segmentation, and analysis. These techniques' novelty is commonly ascertained by three metrics, namely, precision, recall, and F1-Score. The intervention of digital imaging in medical diagnosis has opened up new avenues such as MRI, PET, CT, fMRI, and sMRI.

1.3 ALZHEIMER'S DISEASE

Emil Kraepelin coined Alzheimer's disease (AD) in 1910 in memory of Alois Alzheimer, who initially depicted its symptoms in 1906. This common type of Dementia is otherwise called Dementia of the Alzheimer sort. It is a serious, degenerative, and fatal neuro-disorder which, in general, victimizes individuals of age over and above 65 years of age. According to a recent survey, about 26.6 million individuals worldwide are mentally crippled by this disease. The typical side-effects for this malady are believed to be age-related concerns or stress signs. This disease is characterized by memory loss. The leading cause of Alzheimer's disease is the beta-Amyloid protein. Due to the exponential production or accumulation of a beta-Amyloid protein in the brain, the nerve cells are damaged/ dead. The symptoms of AD are mild memory loss initially, and with an increase in the severity of the disease, patients lose their ability to carry on a conversation and respond to their environment. It is quite cumbersome to diagnose this neurodegenerative disease in its early stages. However, neuroimaging has increased the diagnosis scope, and new standards are prescribed for accurate diagnosis of various brain-related diseases.

The typical stages of degenerations due to AD are -

Stage 1: Slight Memory Loss, Mood Swings, Low response for the actions and slow learning, anxiety of new situations, less energy level.

Stage 2: Discomfort in speaking and comprehension, searching words during a conversation, inability to pay bills, and getting lost while traveling. Further, depression, irritability, and restlessness due to loss of control are also noticed.

Stage 3: The other disorders are short-term memory loss, significant confusions in time, place, and possibly person, para-phasic speech

Stage 4: Incapability to dress correctly, being unaware about the circumstances around them, inability to recall simple details about themselves

Stage 5: Loss of ability to recognize the faces of friends and relatives, inability in bladder and bowel control, significant behavior change.

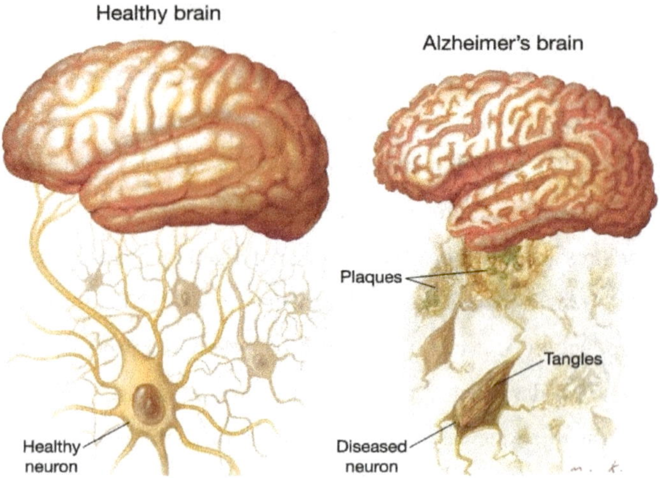

Fig. 1.2 Normal Brain and AD affected Brain

1.4 TYPES OF BRAIN IMAGES

The symptoms of AD are depicted in the sequences of T1-weighted and T2-weighted images. In T1-weighted brain MRI, the Cerebrospinal Fluid (CSF) is darker, whereas, in T2-weighted images, Gray matter appears in high contrast (darker) than the white matter.

1.4.1 T1-Weighted Images

In T1-weighted images, gray matter tissues are presented in dark gray, and white matter tissues are in light gray. The CSF possesses no signal. So, it appears black. T1-weighted MRI on three different orientations are axial, sagittal, and coronal slices, as shown in Fig 1.3

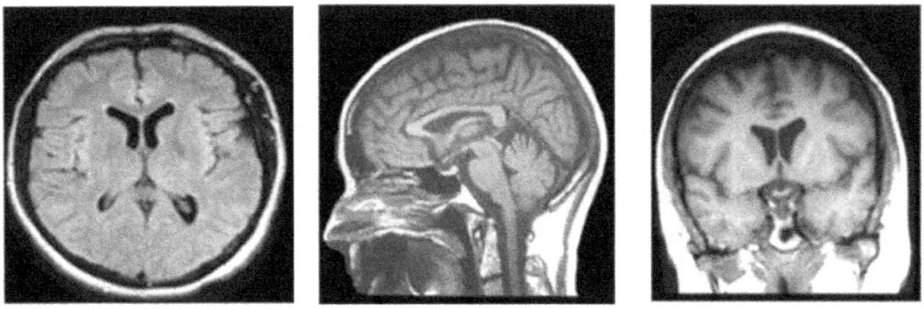

(a) (b) (c)

Fig. 1.3 T1-Weighted Brain Images: (a) Axial Slice (b) Sagittal Slice (c) Coronal Slice

1.4.2 T2-Weighted Images

In T2-weighted images, CSF is brighter, and brain tissues are in the dark. Some T2 sequences possess the additional contrast for gray matter (lighter gray) and white matter (darker gray). T2-weighted MRI on three different orientations are shown in Fig. 1.4

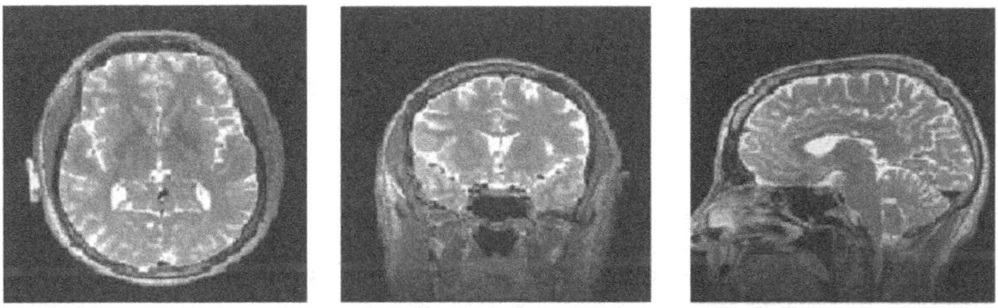

(a) (b) (c)

Fig. 1.4 T2-Weighted Brain Images: (a) Sagittal Slice (b) Coronal Slice (c) Axial Slice

1.5 COMPUTER-AIDED DETECTION

Computer-Aided Detection (CAD) systems can be used to analyze MR brain images and give directions for further diagnosing Alzheimer's disease to physicians. It also evaluates the Alzheimer's areas of density for the MR brain images. Based on the evaluations, the CAD is categorized as Mild Cognitive Impairment (MCI), Front Temporal Dementia (FTD), Very Mild Alzheimer's

Disease (VMAD), and Severe AD that may indicate the shrinkage in brain volume. The CAD is a procedure that helps doctors in the interpretation of medical images. The CAD technology builds from the elements of digital image processing with radiological image analysis. With the help of expert knowledge and image processing techniques, the detection of Alzheimer's Disease has improved impressively. In particular, the CAD system is meant for automated detection and classification of Alzheimer's Disease. This automated detection plays a vital role in the early diagnosis of Alzheimer's Disease.

Structural Magnetic Resonance Imaging (sMRI) scans the internal body structures and also non-invasive imaging techniques. It is mostly used for scanning the brain to visualize the brain's anatomical structures as routine clinical practices. MRI scans facilitate the detailed information of the internal morphological structures of brain tissues such as White Matter (WM), Gray Matter (GM), and Cerebrospinal Fluid (CSF). It also facilitates the facility to identify an image biomarker for AD progression. By recognizing the AD progression, computer-aided diagnosis (CAD) systems are developed using pattern recognition methods.

The image enhancement method enables to improve the visual appearance of images. Image enhancement techniques improve the visual quality of the scan images such as Magnetic Resonance Image (MRI) and Computed Tomography (CT) scan. The Contrast enhancement produces enhanced medical images. The state-of-the-art techniques have the potential to suppress the unwanted noise and enhance the brightness of the images and their contrast. The resulting enhanced medical image provides a pavement for better and easier disease screening process by the radiologists.

1.6 CLASSIFICATION OF MACHINE LEARNING ALGORITHMS

Image classification is the process of extracting the features or attributes from the input images and mark them as classes based on the extracted features/attributes. There are three types of image classification: pixel-wised, sub-pixel-wised, and object-based. This research work focuses on the pixel-wised image classification, categorized as supervised classification, semi-supervised classification, and unsupervised classification.

Machine learning algorithms are classified into three categories, based on their learning capabilities of the learning system *[Kubat, M 2017]* as follows: -

1. **Supervised Learning:** The algorithm creates the model and its predictions by training the example or part of the data. It also processes the actual data with the guidance of the model and predicts the class. The defined model supervises the algorithm's trajectory. The results are produced based on the model's predictions.
2. **Unsupervised Learning:** The algorithm learns from the actual data without any inferences and finds the data patterns on its own. It works based on the features extracted from the data and makes it as classes. These algorithms have no model for giving direction towards the predictions. They learn the identifications of the classes by the features of the images.
3. **Semi-Supervised Learning:** These algorithms are the blend of supervised and unsupervised algorithms. The small portion of the data is adopted for learning by 'model' or 'labeled class,' and the remaining portion is adhered to learn on its own.

The most popular and widely known techniques of machine learning are classification, clustering, and regression.

Classification: This technique aims to classify the input data into different partitions as different classes. It assigns the model or labels to classify and identify the unseen input data based on predicted classes.

Regression: This method is supervised. It predicts the output values based on the labeled predicted values.

Clustering: This is an unsupervised method that classifies the data into different groups without any labeled prediction or model.

Fig. 1.5 shows the types of machine learning classification.

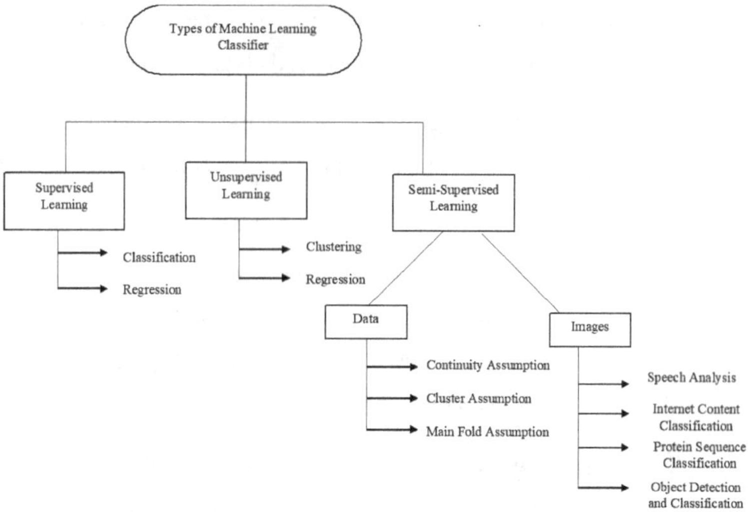

Fig. 1.5 Types of Machine Learning Classification

1.7 CLASSIFICATION OF DEEP LEARNING ALGORITHMS

Deep learning algorithms are the subset of machine learning techniques that facilitate computers to think and do like humans. Deep Learning finds applications in many fields, such as transfer learning, speech, and handwritten character recognition.

In deep learning, the computer learns automatically from the input data and identifies the multiple levels of representations of the data's underlying distribution to be modeled. A deep learning algorithm extracts all the necessary features such as the low and high-level features for classification.

Deep Learning techniques are called as "end-to-end" learning because it gets the raw input image, processes the image, extracts the features, classifies the features and finally, it learns how to do these steps automatically. The features that depend on other features are called 'high level features.

For instance, in the context of computer vision, a deep learning algorithm learns its low level representations such as edge detector, filters, etc., from a raw image and then constructs representations that depend on those low level representations (such as a linear or non-linear combinations of those low-level representations), and successively repeats the same process for higher levels.

The primary advantage of deep learning is automatic representation learning, which improves accuracy, speed, and reduces time consumption than other conventional methods.

1.8 TEST DATASET

1.8.1 Medical Image Dataset

To experiment and estimate the accuracy of our proposed methods, the researcher obtained brain images from the following benchmark datasets.

- Minimal Interval Resonance Imaging in Alzheimer Disease (MIRIAD) [Malone 2013]
- Internet Brain Segmentation Repository (IBSR) [NBSR 2017]
- Open Access Series of Imaging Studies (OASIS)[D. Marcus 2007]

1.8.1.1 MIRIAD Dataset

MIRIAD dataset is a progression of longitudinal volumetric T1 MRI scans of 46 Mild-Moderate Alzheimer's subjects and 23 controls. It is made accessible for specialists to create, approve and look at methods, especially for the estimation of longitudinal volume change in serially acquired MR. Each volume consists of T1-weighted 2D consecutive coronal cuts with measurements of 256 × 256 pixels and the quantity of cuts ranges from 60 to 65 with a cut thickness of 3.1 mm. A few volumes of the dataset had extreme inhomogeneities caused by the non-consistency of attractive fields, radio recurrence curls, and clamor factors [Malone 2013].

1.8.1.2 Internet Brain Segmentation Repository (IBSR) Dataset

The performance of the proposed method was confirmed with twenty volumes of Tl-weighted MR brain images obtained from IBSR of the Centre for Morphometry Analysis (CMA) at the Massachusetts General Hospital. MR brain volumes are obtained from young-middle aged normal individuals. Each volume comprises of 60 to 65 numbers of Tl-weighted 2D sequential coronal slices with dimensions of 256 × 256 pixels with a slice thickness of 3.1 mm [NBSR 2017].

1.8.2 CSV File Dataset

1.8.2.1 Open Access Series of Imaging Studies (OASIS)

The dataset consists of an MRI collection from 416 subjects aged 18 to 96. The MRIs in the collection are cross-sectional images in young, middle-aged, as well as non-demented and demented older adults. The subjects involved come from both genders, and are all right-handed. Out of the 416 subjects, 100 subjects over the age of 60 have been clinically diagnosed with very mild to moderate Alzheimer's disease (AD) [D. Marcus 2007]. The dataset also consists of longitudinal MRI data from 150 non-demented and demented older adults aged 60 to 96. Each of these subjects was scanned on two or more visits with at least one year gap for 373 imaging sessions. Of these, 72 subjects were categorized as non-demented throughout the study; 64 were categorized as demented at the first visit and remained so for subsequent scan sessions, and 51 individuals had mild to moderate Alzheimer's disease. Finally, 14 subjects from this collection were considered as non-demented at their first visit and were characterized later as demented at a later visit. Table 1.1 provides information on the demographics and Table 1.2 provides clinical information.

Table 1.1 Demographics Information

Descriptor	Explanation
M/F	Gender
Hand	Handedness (All subjects were right-handed so that this item can be omitted)
Age	Age in Years
EDUC	Years of Education
SES	Socioeconomic status assessed by the Hollings head Index of Social Position and classified from 1 (highest status) to 5 (lowest status)

Table 1.2 Clinical Information

Descriptor	Explanation
MMSE	Mini-Mental State Examination Score (range is from 0= worst to 30= best)
CDR	Clinical Dementia Rating (0=No dementia, 0.5 = very mild AD, 1=mild AD, 2 =moderate AD)

1.9 METRICS FOR PERFORMANCE ANALYSIS

The performance of the proposed method and the existing method are measured by using the similarity measure Jaccard (J) and Dice (D). These methods will take two images as input and produce the value between 0 and 1.

The Jaccard [Wagner, J 2012] value is calculated by:

$$J(S_1, S_2) = \frac{|S_1 \cap S_2|}{|S_1 \cup S_2|} \tag{1.1}$$

The Dice [Wagner, J 2012] value is measured by:

$$D(S_1, S_2) = \frac{2|S_1 \cap S_2|}{|S_1| + |S_2|} \tag{1.2}$$

The level of accuracy makes the results of the devised methodology as acceptable. The evaluation metric is a very important feature for the performance assessment of the classifier model [2019]. In Table 1.3 and Table 1.4, the confusion matrix demonstrates the results of incorrectly and correctly classified instances of each class in the three classes of the problem.

The accuracy is a commonly used evaluation metric. Other metrics include the following.

$$Precision = \frac{tp}{(tp+fp)} \tag{1.3}$$

$$Recall = \frac{tp}{(tp+fn)} \tag{1.4}$$

$$F1 - Measure = \frac{(1+\beta)^2 * Recall * Precision}{\beta^2 * Recall * Precision} \tag{1.5}$$

where β is a co-efficient to adjust the importance of precision and recall (usually β =1)

$$FP_{rate} = \frac{FP}{(FP+TN)} \quad (1.6)$$

$$TP_{rate} = \frac{TP}{(TP+FN)} \quad (1.7)$$

Table 1.3 Elements of Confusion Matrix

Descriptor	Explanation
True Positive (TP)	Classifier predicted the test samples as diseased when they have the disease
True Negative (TN)	Classifier predicted no disease when they don't have the disease
False Positive (FP)	Classifier predicted the test samples as diseased, but they don't have the disease
False Negative (FN)	Classifier predicted no disease, but they have the disease

Table 1.4 Metrics from Confusion Matrix

Descriptor	Explanation
Accuracy	(TP + TN)
Misclassification Rate	(FP + FN)=Total
True Positive Rate or Recall	TP=Actual Yes
False Positive Rate	FP=Actual No = 10=60
True Negative Rate	TN=Actual No = 50=600:83

These metrics have been used on the output of various tested MRI Alzheimer's Disease better performance, and high accuracy is achieved for all the tested normal and AD affected MR brain images.

1.10 OBJECTIVES OF THE RESEARCH

The major objectives, given below, form the framework of the research work:

- To develop novel algorithms to
  - remove the artifacts present in the input MR brain images.
  - extract the brain parts using on the Region of Interest (RoI)
- Segment WM and GM from the MR brain images to distinguish between normal and abnormal brain tissues.
- Detect the presence and absence of AD and categorize AD into the respective stage, based on its severity.

1.11 OUTLINE OF THE RESEARCH

This research has brought out nine distinct strategies: pre-processing, WM and GM segmentation, data analysis and classification of MRI AD analysis, and categorization of Healthy Control brain images.

I. **Pre-Processing of MR Brain Images**
   (a) Threshold Based Extraction of Brain Parts
   (b) Rician noise removal of PSMF filter
   (c) Data Imputation based classification

II. **White Matter and Gray Matter Segmentation from MRI Brain Images**
   (a) Expectation-Maximization and k-Means Clustering-based Segmentation

III. **Multi-Class classification using Machine Learning Algorithms**
   (a) Alzheimer's disease classification using Gradient Processing Classifier with Hyper parameter Tuning (GPC-HPT) model.
   (b) Alzheimer's disease classification using Decision Tree Classifier with Hyper parameter Tuning (AD-DTC-HPT).

(c) Alzheimer's disease classification using an Ensemble of Logistic Regression Models with Hyperparameter Tuning (AD-ELR-HPT) model.

IV. Analysis of Alzheimer's Disease using Deep Learning

(a) Alzheimer's disease analysis using Convolutional Neural Network (CNN)

(b) Alzheimer's disease analysis using Optimized Transfer Learning (OTL)

1.12 ORGANIZATION OF THE THESIS

This thesis is organized into nine chapters, as described below:

1. Introduction
2. Review of Literature
3. Pre-Processing of MR Brain Images
4. MR Brain Image Segmentation Methods
5. Multinomial Logistic Regression Model for Classification of Alzheimer's Disease
6. Enhanced Tree-Based Classifier for Effective Classification of Alzheimer's Disease
7. Ensemble Based Classification of Alzheimer's Disease
8. Optimized Convolutional Neural Network for AD Classification
9. Summary of Conclusions

Chapter 1 describes the fundamentals of Medical Image Processing, MRI, Alzheimer's Disease, Classification using machine learning and deep learning as well as diagnosis of AD. The scope and objectives of the thesis are given in this section.

A detailed review of region-based segmentation and classification of Alzheimer's disease in MR brain images are given in Chapter 2. The research gap elicited out of the literature review is explained in this chapter.

Chapter 3 describes novel pre-processing methods for MR brain images, namely Threshold-based Morphological Operations and Artifacts Removal (TMOAR), Rician noise removal based on Progressive Median Switching Filter (PMSF). The data imputation on clinical data is also performed for data cleaning.

Chapter 4 describes intensity-based segmentation methods, namely Thresholded and Morphological operation based Brain Segmentation (TMOS) and MR Brain Image Segmentation using k-Means Clustering and Expectation Maximization (MRB-kM-EM). The TMOS proposes a Region-based technique using skull removal. The MRB-kM-EM segments WM and GM segmentation using Healthy Control (HC) and AD brain images, which results in precise segmentation. These methods form a framework for brain tissue segmentation using optimal localization of Region of Interest (RoI).

Chapter 5 presents the methodology, metrics, and merits of AD Classification using Multinomial Logistic Regression (MNLR). A comparative analysis of MNLR over the conventional Multinomial Logistic classifier model is given in this chapter.

Chapter 6 explains the implementation of the Gradient Boosting Classifier (GBC) and Decision Tree Classifier with Hyper parameter tuning (DTC). The performance analysis of these methods is given in this chapter.

Chapter 7 explains the procedure and performance of Ensemble-based Classifier (EC) and Random Forest Classifier with Hyper parameter tuning (RFC-HPT). The proposed methods are tested on the clinical data drawn from OASIS dataset.

Chapter 8 explains the methodology of Optimized Convolutional Neural Network (AD-OCNN) and Optimized Transfer Learning (AD-OTL) models designed for this research are reported in Chapter 8. The MR brain images taken from MIRIAD dataset are used for the validation of results

Chapter 9 summarizes the conclusions of the reported research work. The future directions for this research work are also given in this chapter.

This research work has brought out optimal and feasible solutions for Alzheimer's Disease detection and classification using the principles of traditional, machine learning and Deep Learning computational methods. The improved accuracy depicted by the proposed methods endorses the objectives of this research. These reported techniques can be suitably deployed in the development of an automated Alzheimer's detection and classification system, which forms scope of future research.

CHAPTER 2

REVIEW OF LITERATURE

Alzheimer's Disease (AD) is a progressive neural disorder, causing the degeneration of physical and mental activities, particularly among the old age groups. It gets worsened from time to time due to the brain cell's degeneration, causing shrinkage in the brain's volume.

During Image acquisition, the captured image may get corrupted with Rician noise, Gaussian noise, and impulse noise. Hence it is mandatory to suppress the respective noise as a pre-processing step. Image segmentation deals with the extraction of discrete objects or components of a given image. The machine learning and deep learning techniques were explored to review their potential and applicability in the detection or diagnosis of AD.

This chapter summarizes the prominent research contributions on the essential domains, namely noise removal, segmentation, machine learning, and deep learning techniques.

2.1 NOISE REMOVAL METHODS

Aja-Fernández et al. (2008) developed a method for the localization of targeted regions in the given MRI images using its local statistics, namely local variance, local mean, and Linear Minimum Mean Square Error (LMMSE). The dynamic estimation of noise is computed using recursive LMMSE. The performance of this method produced better noise removal potential and better feature preservation.

Sarode et al. (2010) proposed the Rician noise suppression method. This method showed that the Rician noise suppression rate is appreciable. Their algorithm has exhibited promising results on complex MR images.

Devasena et al. (2011) developed a novel hybrid filter method to reduce random noise in MR images by combining Kernel, Sobel, and Low-pass filtering (KSL) techniques. This method is implemented in Matlab and compared with the related state of art methods regarding the synthetic and real clinical MR images. The KSL shows superior performance in all those cases taken for evaluation.

Balafar M. A (2012) has critically reviewed noise reduction techniques for brain images and presented the advantages and disadvantages of noise reduction techniques. Moreover, the comparative study of the different noise reduction techniques is listed. *Koli M.A et al.* (2012) discussed the survey of impulse noise reduction techniques. The research work performs a comparison of ten popular techniques of impulse noise reduction techniques. The results of all those methods were analyzed, and the efficiency of those algorithms is also reported. *Sajjad Mohsin et al.* (2012) proposed an improved noise reduction technique that produces robust, accurate, and fully automated skull-stripping methods.

Kumar B.S et al. (2013) described a Non-Local Means Filter and its Noise Thresholding Method (NLFTM) to remove noise and preserve edge details. Discrete Wavelet Transform (DWT) presents the phenomenon of Gibbs at the subtle edge of tissue. Jangra et al. (2014) have improved denoising Rician noise reduction using the principle of wave atom shrinkage. Zhang et al. (2014) have modified the Recursive Non-Local Mean (RNLM) filter into RNLM-CPP, where CPP stands for Combined Patch Pixel. The RNLM-CPP filter results on synthetic and real MR brain images produced a better performance and preserved small and high contrast particle information than its predecessor.

Shrestha et al. (2014) have compared a few denoising techniques and suggested a unique method for removing impulse noise using the decision-based strategy. These techniques, while suppressing impulse noise, mainly retained image information. Mean Square Error (MSE) and Peak Signal to Noise Ratio (PSNR) of various filtered images depict those techniques' merits. The researchers have also validated the results, esteems with visual perception.

Yang et al. (2015) developed a pre-smooth Non-Local Means (NLM) filter for MRI brain images, combined with image transformation. They experimented with the NLM filter with weights calculated from the pre-smoothed images on the transformed MRI. They further applied an inverse transformation operation and restored the denoised MRI. A combination of NLM and Stationary Wavelet Transform (SWT) with adaptive thresholds was developed by Jeevakala et al. (2016) to remove Rician noise and maintain structural data such as edges of the image. This technique produced better results than other denoising techniques.

The MR brain images created by Renukalatha S et al. (2016) are generally corrupted by Rician noise, which would mislead image analysis algorithms and result in incorrect disease diagnosis. Poorly depicted tumor boundaries would be an obstacle for subsequent tumor analysis, such as the extraction of features, classification, and quantification.

Biswas et al. (2018) developed a new noise removal method used with curvelet transform thresholding, combined with the Wiener filter, for the Magnetic Brain Resonance Imaging (MRI). They compared the result with other denoising techniques based on curvelet and wavelet. Peak-Signal-Noise-Ratio (PSNR), Mean Square Error (MSE), and Structural Similarity (SSIM) were used to evaluate the quality of the image. The results of the experiment show that their method shows better results than their competitors.

Suhas S et al. (2018) developed the Gaussian, Max, Min, and Medium Arithmetic filters. Those filters are applied to the MR brain images and spinal cord. The output image's effectiveness is evaluated by statistical parameters such as root-mean-square error (RMSE) and signal-to-noise ratios (SNR), the PSNR.

Murugan et al. (2018) developed a hybrid multi-resolution filter that indicates degraded MR brain images with salt and pepper noises and incorporates the transformation wavelet to improve its resolution. The hybrid filter consists of a three-value weighted filter and a resemblance-based filter. A local variable window is used to spot the noisy pixels in a three-value weighted filter. The intensity of the noise-free pixels in the window is used to reconstruct corrupted pixels. A variable local window for rebuilding noisy pixels are used in a similarity-based filter.

Roy et al. (2018) developed a k-Means based method that divides a corrupted image into a vector set, and the corresponding function vectors are built with 10 %, 50 %, and the impulse sound of 90%. In testing phases, the pixel is shown as noisy; the histogram adaptive fuzzy filter will be used over the noisy pixels. It is noted that efficiency is improved approximately 2-5 dB compared to baseline filters that are likely to be SVM fuzzy filters and an adaptive mean filter (ANNASMF) based on artificial neural network.

Damini et al. (2019) discussed noise reduction techniques on medical images. The Non-Local Means (NLM) filter and other kinds of Rician noise in MR brain images are also discussed. NLM improves textures and borders of an image. The NLM filter is a practicable technique to reduce geometrical setup by achieving the least outcomes.

Divya S et al. (2019) reported on the alternative MR brain image denoising procedures in spatial, transform, and machine learning domains. This method performed better than its counterparts in noise reduction, boundary preservation, robustness, user interaction, computation, complexity, and cost.

Brain MRIs are corrupted with different noises, namely, Rician noise, Gaussian noise, Salt and Pepper noise, that call for noise suppression. The scope for improvement in noise suppression and edge or detail preservation confirms the need to develop newer noise reduction methods.

2.2 MR BRAIN IMAGE SEGMENTATION METHODS

Capelle et al. (2003) proposed a 3D segmentation of multi-echo MR brain images into White Matter (WM), Gray Matter (GM), and Cerebrospinal Fluid (CSF) by using the fusion process, based on the evidence theory and also add the neighborhood information knowledge to get more accurate and efficient results. Wang et al. (2008) have suggested using a novel dissimilarity index instead of the usual distance metrics to apply both local and non-local data in the conventional Fuzzy C-Means (FCM) clustering algorithm. It is proved that the obtained results are better than the reported one.

Kannan et al. (2009) proposed a novel FCM algorithm for MR brain image segmentation, using weighted bias estimation. In this method, the objective function of the conventional algorithm has been modified and implemented. Even the brain images with inhomogeneous intensities and different image noises, this technique generated excellent outcomes.

FCM failed to segment image properly due to homogeneity, low contrast, noise, and content inequality with semantic, automatic techniques. Balafar et al. (2010) suggested a technique using fast FCM to enhance image efficiency. The volumetric structural modifications were evaluated with both brains GM and WM in dyslexic adolescents. In cerebella, GM, and WM, patients with MSA-C (Multiple System Atrophy-Cerebellum) showed a reduced fractal dimension (FD) that suggests cerebellar structure degeneration. The segmentation of the nerve tissue also allows for the diagnosis of nerve tissue illnesses.

Wu YT et al. (2010) developed a new scalp, skull, CSF GM, and WM segmentation technique in mouse brain MRI based on a threshold, k-means Clustering, and narrow-band level set techniques.

The amygdale helps in the early detection of AD, which causes neuropsychiatric symptoms to the patients. Ito et al. (2011) proposed using unsupervised neural networks such as a self-organizing map and fuzzy adaptive theory to segment the brain tissue, and the results reveal CSF and tissue segmentation compared to FCM. Therefore, the AD is detected, and the exact location is identified. The level set approach for image segmentation is proposed by Li C et al. (2011). The sensitivity and accuracy of brain regions' structural features were thoroughly studied for early AD diagnosis by Knafo et al. (2012).

Zivadinov et al. (2012) reported that studies on multiple sclerosis and the gray matter pathology are on the rise. Myelin sheath is extensively damaged when there is multiple sclerosis. Zanaty et al. (2012) provided a hybrid strategy to evaluate the gray matter and white matter tissue in brain MRI using fuzzy clustering, seed area growth, and Jacquard similarity coefficient algorithms. This technique operates well on anatomical data intensity values. First, the brain image was split into distinct regions, and then a seed point for the increasing seed region growing method is employed to segment brain tissues.

Mohsin et al. (2012) suggested an enhanced method that generated robust, precise, and an automated skull removal compared to a few other pre-processing techniques to support an area of interest. Charulatha et al. (2013) evaluated the clustering method using an FCM with five different distance measures. For the diagnosis of multiple brain-related illnesses caused due to the modifications or damage to the brain. Kaushik et al. (2013) segmented white matter from brain MR images to segment the brain images' nerve tissues using segmentation principles.

Patel et al. (2014) proposed an adaptive clustering technique that automatically selected the cluster value and combined the pixels of similar intensities to a form of the designated region(s). The level set method was used applied to smoothen the segmented regions.

Tembhekar et al. (2015) developed a Spatial K-Fuzzy Clustering Method (SKFCM) for image segmentation. This algorithm provided an approximate boundary and applied level set after clustering that yielded the exact boundary of white matter, gray matter, and Cerebrospinal fluid.

Ali et al. (2015) proposed MR brain image segmentation consisting of three processes. The multi-resolution wavelet decomposition is applied to maintain the spatial context between the pixels. Then, the morphological pyramid fusion technique increases the image's sharpness and reduces the image's noise. Finally, the Fuzzy C-Means clustering technique is applied for segmentation. Despotovic et al. (2015) described that segmentation is widely used to measure and visualize anatomical brain structures for surgical planning and image-guided interventions. They have proposed various segmentation methods to address the complexity, challenges, and validation of MRI brain segmentation.

Deepa et al. (2015) suggested a useful technique for automatic segmentation from MR brain images of gray matter and white matter regions using Fuzzy C-Means and Kohonen Means Clustering techniques. Based on the intensity values and statistical characteristics, the gray matter and white matter are segmented. A technique based on binarization, wavelet decomposition, and the convex hull was suggested by Roy et al. (2015) and generated acceptable results. It is tested on three distinct types of MR brain images (Transverse, Sagital, and Coronal), and experiment validation suggests accurate detection and segmentation of morphological structures or a specific region of MR brain images. Martinez M.F.J et al. (2016) described techniques that perform spherical brain mapping to detect the AD by projecting the three-dimensional MRI brain images into two-dimensional maps measurements that reveal the tissue's statistical characteristics.

Gnana J. D et al. (2017) developed a new mechanism for white matter segmentation from MRI brain image. The proposed method is a hybrid approach that sequentially performs artifacts removal, noise suppression, and contrast enhancement followed by k- means based segmentation. This method showed a mean of 87% Dice Similarity Index (DSI) with a standard deviation of ± 5.74 against the manual segmentation shown as ground truth. The experiment was performed on T1-MRIs.

Xiao et al. (2017) developed a novel method to combine three distinct structural MR brain image features: gray-matter volume, gray-level matrix co-occurrence, and Gabor feature. These characteristics can obtain both 2D and 3D brain data, and the experimental findings have shown that better performance can be achieved through multi-feature fusion. The suggested feature selection algorithm could effectively extract the optimal characteristics subset to improve the classification effectiveness.

Mito, R et al. (2018) designed a novel method known as pixel-based assessment that comprehensively explored the variations among the voxels, estimate the axonal losses due to Alzheimer's disease and mild cognitive impairment. The authors hypothesized that patients with Alzheimer's disease would display comprehensive functional degeneration.

Zhang T et al. (2018) developed two Fuzzy Clustering algorithm optimization solutions based on the Local Gaussian likelihood Fuzzy C-means (LGP-FCM) model and Anisotropic Weight Fuzzy C-means (AW-FCM) model and applied it on the brain MRI for segmentation.

Kong Z et al. (2019) suggested a wavelet-based method to capture the distinct contours. The automatic segmentation of the image can be done using the CNN model with deep learning. The segmented gray and white matter information is quantified to indicate this segmentation technology's ability to quantitatively diagnose cerebral atrophy.

2.3 MACHINE LEARNING BASED SEGMENTATION

In the medical field, automated diagnosis of brain disorder with MR images is becoming increasingly essential. Several works are provided below linked to the classification of AD. Some significant research contributions of Machine Learning based segmentation are reported here is under. Due to the latest technological advancements in big data and artificial intelligence, the research contributions on machine learning are rising.

Freund et al. (1997) reported the learning aspect and the generic decision-theoretical method's applications. In boosting, the authors implemented a multiplicative weight update process and evaluated it in the light of learning algorithms and features. Chaplot et al. (2006) proposed a mechanism that can transform MR brain images into wavelets into Self Organizing Map (SOM) inputs. These MR brain pictures are classified as either normal or abnormal. This research offers better precision on classification. Moreover, some have outperformed SVM.

El-Dahshan E.S.A et al. (2010) presented a tri-phase AD classifier for MRIs that combines the extracted features, dimensionality reduction for AD classification. For the extraction of features, they used Discrete Wavelet Transformation (DWT), Principle Component Analysis (PCA) for feature reduction, Feed-Forward back-Propagation Artificial Neural Network (FP-

ANN), and k-nearest neighbour (k-NN) for classification. The accuracy of classification by those methods was 97% or above.

Joshi S et al. (2010) developed a multi-layer perceptron, bagging, decision tree, Co-active Neuro-Fuzzy Inference System (CANFIS), and genetic algorithm that have been created using distinct machine learning techniques for AD classification. The CANFIS method's classification precision was 99.55 %. Claudia Plant et al. (2010) created a hybrid model to detect brain atrophy trends and predict Alzheimer's disease, using SVM and Bayesian Classifier. It produced a corresponding pattern index of 92%.

Ye J et al. (2011) explained the causes and consequences of AD and have used multi-source data fusion and multi-source biomarkers for neuroimaging detection. This research utilized Sparse Inverse Covariance Estimation (SICE)-based methods to find connectivity and its strength. They developed a machine learning-based multi-modal data fusion for medical images. Hamou et al. (2011) suggested a cluster analysis method for AD diagnosis from MR based images.

A supervised approach was used by Filipovych R et al. (2012) to classify images using the SVM model. A new methodology was created by Herrera L J et al. (2013) to classify MR brain pictures into ordinary, and AD influenced pictures. Their technique is emphasized by the extraction of MRI features in the wavelet domain, followed by a decrease of dimensionality and the classification of SVM. The diagnosis of AD was recorded by Escudero J et al. (2013) using machine learning methods. Lebedev et al. (2014) have created Computer-Aided Design for AD.

Li et al. (2015) proposed a modification of classical deep learning strategy for AD diagnosis using images from MRI, and the authors had investigated the dropout impact as a solution for handling overfitting, induced by weighing co-adaptation. They suggested a new deep learning structure infused with the choice of stability, adaptive learning, and multitask learning to classify input images into AD Mild Cognitive Impairment (MCI). This research verified that integrating dropout into deep learning increases classification precision.

Sampath et al. (2015) developed a new image segmentation and fMRI AD detection technique. For the extraction and segmentation of features, this work used Network, and the Adaptive Neuro-Fuzzy Inference System (ANFIS) was used for classification. This combinatorial strategy for AD detection yielded significant outcomes.

Li et al. (2015) proposed a new approach based on Principle Component Analysis (PCA). It uses the permanence selection and dropout models, and the Restricted Boltzmann Machine (RBM) model, a deep learning approach.

Tohka et al. (2016) comparatively analyzed SVM's performance and features-based classification algorithms that detect the level of dementia using fMRI datasets. This work reported on the classification of AD and MCI against Normal Control (NC) by using split-half re-sampling from the Alzheimer's Disease Neuroimaging (ADNI) database. The study focused on the impact of feature selection with and without a filter and embedded features against SVM. The study concluded that the selection of sample size and the number of features substantially influence classification accuracy.

Lama R.K et al. (2017) summarize the advantages of machine learning techniques to detect AD in neuroimaging, namely, PET, MRI, and Fluoro Deoxy Glucose (FDG) PET scan. The authors indicate that functional brain connectivity observations can ideally identify and diagnose AD and classify the input images as MCI and Healthy Control (HC). The principles used include SVM, Import Vector Machine (IVM), and Regularized Extreme Learning Machine (RELM). This work also includes developing another classification mechanism exclusively for complex datasets, using the ADNI database for experimental analysis. Balamurgan M *et al.* (2017) designed a dimensionality reduction technique based on the KNN classification algorithm. This method is used to analyze and classify the AD and MCI. This classification model gives better results in the form of higher accuracy and sensitivity.

Bi X.A et al. (2018) proposed the random neural system group to enhance the order of execution. The dataset for their experimentation was selected from the ADNI. The Elman Neural Network was confirmed to be an ideal base classifier that utilizes the arbitrary neural system cluster, which is dependent on the outcome of highlighted selections, with an accuracy of 92.31%. Bi *et al.* (2018) used a random support vector machine clustering to diagnose AD and group the disease regions into the inferior frontal gyrus, superior frontal gyrus, precentral gyrus, and cingulate cortex.

Wang Z et al. (2018) developed a new method name as Resting-State fMRI Based Network Connectivity Analysis (RS-fMRINC) for feature vector-based classification for AD detection.

Tzimourta K D et al. (2019) have reported a study for detecting AD over different brain regions. This technique can detect AD from Electron Encephalogram (EEG) using several statistical and spectral features. The accuracy of the region model is ranged from 88% to 96% for whole-brain classification. Moore P.J et al. (2019) developed a new method with a random forest classifier to predict AD. This model used a pairwise selection from time-series data. The data analysis obtained from the random forest classifier algorithm was used to learn the relationship between pairs of data points.

Das D. et al. (2019) proposed a new approach named "Sparse High-order Interaction Model with Rejection option (SHIMR)". This interpretable SHIMR uses a weighted sum of short rules that are tested on 151 data taken from Alzheimer's Disease Neuroimaging Initiative (ADNI). It has exhibited sensitivity and specificity of about 0.84 and 0.69 respectively.

2.4 DEEP LEARNING BASED METHODS

Automated brain disorder diagnosis with MR images has become increasingly important in the medical. Image classification can detect and categorize abnormal images into different groups. The summary of review given in this research covers the traditional methods and deep learning approaches for AD diagnosis.

Zhang D et al. (2011) proposed a multi-kernel SVM to enhance the classification's efficiency. A deep learning framework based on 3D Convolutional Neural Networks (CNN) has been suggested to estimate missing PET imaging information for MRI information. Then the MRI Voxel-wise gray matter density map and PET intensity values are coupled with a sparse regression classifier for multi-modal AD classification.

Bhagya Shree S R et al. (2014) discussed the different neuropsychological tests' review, the different diagnostic algorithms used for the analysis.

Sarraf S et al. (2016) introduced a unique technique of classifying Alzheimer's brain from a normal healthy brain using CNN. The significance of medical dataset classification is to possibly build a model or mechanism of prediction to identify or diagnose the disease from the clinical dataset and categorize it into the respective stages. The classification of clinical information such as AD has always been challenging, and selecting the most discriminatory features has always been the most challenging part. They used CNN and the renowned LeNet-5 architecture for AD diagnosis. The accuracy was 98% on brain MRI of normal controls. This experiment proposed that the invariant shift and scale features obtained by CNN and deep learning classification are the most efficient techniques for distinguishing clinical information from healthy fMRI information.

Ortiz A et al. (2016) developed the classification methods based on deep learning architectures and applied to brain regions defined by the Automated Anatomical Labeling (AAL). Gray Matter (GM) images from each brain region were divided into 3D patches according to the areas defined by the AAL atlas and these patches are used to train various deep neural networks. Then, an ensemble of deep belief networks is comprised in which a voting system determines the final prediction. Two deep learning-based models and four different voting systems are introduced and compared, resulting in powerful classification architecture that computes discriminative features in an unsupervised manner. The classification architecture specifically offers accuracy values of up to 90% and 95%. The Area under Receiver Operating Characteristics (ROC) Area Under the Curve (AUC) for Normal Control (NC) / AD classification, 84% and 91% AUC for stable MCI / AD classification and 83% and AUC of 95% for NC/MCI converters classification.

A novel technique to diagnosing AD was created by Ju R (2017) based on profound neural networks and various medical data. Model training and classification of fMRI images and text, including year, gender, and genetic information, are performed.

Gulhare K K et al. (2017) presented a new approach for Alzheimer's disease detection through Deep Neural Network (DNN) classification. The longitudinal MRI information was used in the non-demented and demented older adult dataset. An image segmentation mechanism tagged with the selection of attributes was designed. Finally, classification using the DNN is implemented for the detection of AD. The DNN properly-recognized AD with an accuracy of 96.6% and the minimum error rate is obtained.

Luo S et al. (2017) developed a new method for automatic recognition of AD using a deep learning model. It used CNN based classification using 3D brain images. The innovation was qualified and experienced based on MRI data from the ADNI dataset. The findings showed that the higher sensitivity detection of AD accuracy is 100% and 93% specificity.

Lu D et al. (2018) explored a new technique to enhance the novel deep learning-based approach's efficiency. This method produced with 82% accuracy in identifying individuals with MCI who may convert and get to AD at three years before conversion (86.4% combined conversion accuracy within 1–3 years), 94% sensitivity in classifying individuals with probable AD clinical diagnosis, and 86% specificity in classifying non-demented controls.

Liu J (2018) developed an efficient whole-brain hierarchical network to extract features for MRI-based classification of AD. The hierarchical network used the texture features of ROI for better classification accuracy. This method also provided the high-dimension features obtained from raw feature spaces during AD classification by computing the features' F-score. A Multiple Kernel Classifier (MK-C) improved the classification performance on the images. The experimental results on the MRI data from the ADNI database show that this proposed method is efficient and is promising for clinical applications for AD diagnosis.

Lohar M.V (2018) presented a new approach for the automatic classification procedure for the detection of Alzheimer's disease, with the main focus on enhancing predictive accuracy that was helpful for AD detection practitioners and their progression phases such as NC, MCI, and AD. This study of the latest research aimed at semi-or fully automatic computer-assisted AD progression diagnosis.

Awate G et al. (2018) proposed a new method for detecting Alzheimer's Disease from MRI using CNN with the Tensor flow using the transfer learning model. This model has classified the various stages of AD. Islam J et al. (2018) designed a new method, namely AD diagnosis, using the ensemble of deep CNN models. These models are used for the clinical dataset to identify the different stages of AD for early diagnosis.

Cheng B et al. (2018) have developed a novel transfer learning method for early AD analysis. A robust multi-label transfer learning model was generated by this method.

Sajna T et al. (2018) developed a new method for the two-stage CNN model prediction for early AD diagnosis. The image patches were taken as input to learning inherent associations between local image patches and target landmarks in the first stage. In the second stage, the entire image is taken as input, and finally, it detects AD.

Liu J et al. (2018) designed a deep learning application for MRI images that offers an extensive overview of MRI images' processing and analysis. Xiaoheng Tan X et al. (2018) have developed a new three-stage framework technique. First, the transfer of gravity deals with the source domain nearer to the destination data set. Second, the highest deviation between the transmitted source domain samples and the target domain samples are searched using wrapper-based Instance Transfer learning (ITL) algorithm to obtain optimally transferred domain samples. Finally, for classification, those samples are combined with the target domain training samples.

Zhou K et al. (2018) introduced a new approach for feature selection and transferred learning for clinical diagnosis of Alzheimer's disease. The MR images were segmented using the spm-Dartel toolbox and recorded with the atlas Automatic Anatomical Labeling (AAL). Then the volume of the anatomical gray matter region was measured as a characteristic parameter. It has used information gain for the feature selection.

Wu C et al. (2018) developed the Deep Convolutional Neural Networks (DCNNs) that were adopted for distinguishing the different stages of MCI from the NC group and predict the time of conversion from MCI to AD. Two CNN architectures, including GoogleNet and CaffeNet, have been explored and evaluated using transfer learning from pre-trained ImageNet.

Usama M et al. (2018) established a new multi-modal risk assessment model based on Recurrent Convolutional Neural Network (RCNN) using structured and unstructured data. By using the recurrent intra-layer link, the CNN layer becomes a bidirectional RNN. Each neuron within the convolutional layer collects feed-forward and recurrent inputs respectively from the prior unit and neighbourhood. The predictive accuracy of the model is 96%.

For a smart diagnosis of Alzheimer's disease, Razavi, F et al. (2019) suggested that machine learning methods, particularly deep learning, were considered helpful for learning raw data features. A two-layer uncontrolled neural network was used at the first stage of learning, scattered faltering, to learn features from raw data directly. Based on the learned features, Softmax regression was used in the second phase to categorize the health status. The technique proposed was validated by Alzheimer's Brain Images datasets.

Huang, Y et al. (2019) developed a new CNN based technique to integrate all the multi-modality information included in the hippocampus area's T1-MR and FDG-PET images for AD diagnosis. Unlike traditional machine learning algorithms, this technique does not involve manually extracted features; instead, it uses 3D image processing CNNs to learn AD diagnosis or prognosis features.

Lee G et al. (2019) developed a new system integrating multi-domain longitudinal data. The prediction model for MCI transformation to AD provided accuracy of up to 75% (area under curve (AUC) = 0.83) with only one modality of data separately and this prediction model achieved. The performance by 81% accuracy (AUC=0.86) with incorporating longitudinal multi-domain data. A multi-modal deep learning approach has the potential to identify the subjects at risk of developing AD.

Awate G. (2018) proposed a new method for detecting AD from MRI using CNN using transfer learning and the BellCNN model. This model uses two stages: The first stage is Transfer Learning Model applied to ADNI dataset images, and the second stage is BellCNN that refers to the respective CNN and its classification based on the various stages of AD.

Ju R et al. (2019) designed the brain network using Resting-state Functional Magnetic Resonance Imaging (R-fMRI) data to calculate brain regions' functional connectivity. A targeted autoencoder network is constructed to differentiate the normal aging cases from mild cognitive impairment. The technique efficiently shows discriminative brain network features and provides a reliable AD detection classifier. The proposed deep learning technique accomplishes about 31% improvement in prediction accuracy, and the standard deviation decreases by 51%. In the best case, that means this prediction model is more stable and reliable compared to the traditional methods.

2.5 RESEARCH GAP

The literature review gives an account of various techniques devised for the classification of MR Brain Images for AD detection. The pitfalls in those techniques highlight the greater scope for the development of better computational solutions. It is evident that, in addition to segmentation, feature extraction, and classification, the medical image processing system must have the computational capability for pre-processing viz., noise suppression, and region localization. The computational procedures reported in the literature, namely, Maximum Likelihood, Artificial Neural Network (ANN), Decision Trees, Bayesian Classifier, SVM, despite the advantages, are constrained by the respective principal components, viz., dependence on accuracy and model parameters. The emergence of new strategies, such as meta-heuristic techniques, augments computational intelligence, and outcomes. The feature-based classification and prediction techniques are proven to possess ample scope for the early diagnosis of AD patterns. These factors motivated the researcher to develop new strategies for MR brain image classification for Alzheimer's Disease.

CHAPTER 3

PRE-PROCESSING OF MR BRAIN IMAGES

3.1 INTRODUCTION

Magnetic Resonance Imaging (MRI) is the most reliable and widely used source for detecting abnormalities. The interpretation of the results of brain analysis primarily requires the expertise of radiologists and medical practitioners. This lead to the development of many Computer-Aided Detection (CAD) methods for the automatic detection and analysis of Alzheimer's Disease (AD). The captured brain images are influenced by noise, unwanted labels, and artifacts. [Latha M et al., 2019].

3.2 MR IMAGES

Medical imaging is used to study the internal organs' structure, thereby diagnosing and treating various diseases [Dong, Z 2015]. Magnetic Resonance Imaging (MRI) of the brain can assist in identifying specific ailments or chronic neural disorders/ diseases. In this section, the anatomy of the human brain s described.

3.3 HUMAN BRAIN ANATOMY

The human brain is a vital regulatory organ that controls and manages the voluntary and involuntary actions of a human body. The skull protects the brain, and it comprises three main components of the brain, temporal lobe, and cerebellum, as depicted in Fig. 3.1. The brainstem functions as the core for the spinal cord relay between the cerebrum and the cerebellum.

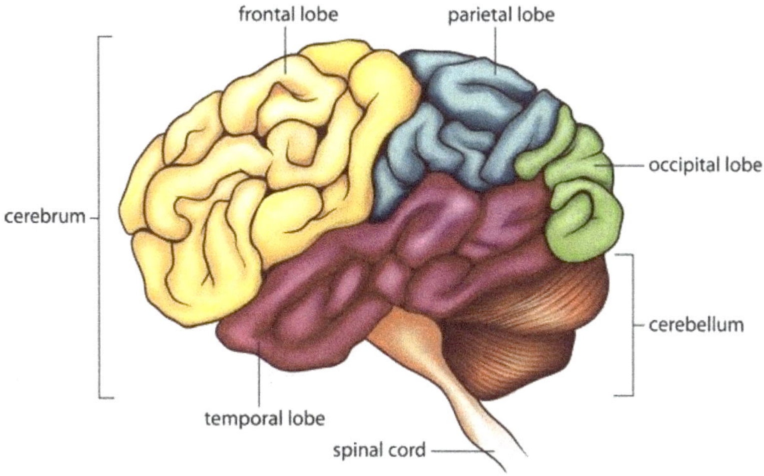

Fig. 3.1 Human Brain Anatomy

3.4 MR BRAIN IMAGE SEGMENTATION

The image pre-processing stage aims to improve the images' quality and make them suitable for the subsequent phase of image processing.

Hence, the pre-processing stage of this research study contains three phases that aim to develop newer strategies to

- Labels/ artifacts removal
- Noise removal in brain image
- Data Imputation

The first phase entails removing unwanted information from the brain images, and the second phase deals with the suppression of noise such as Rician, Gaussian, and impulse noise in MR brain images. The overall research framework for AD classification is given in Fig. 3.2.

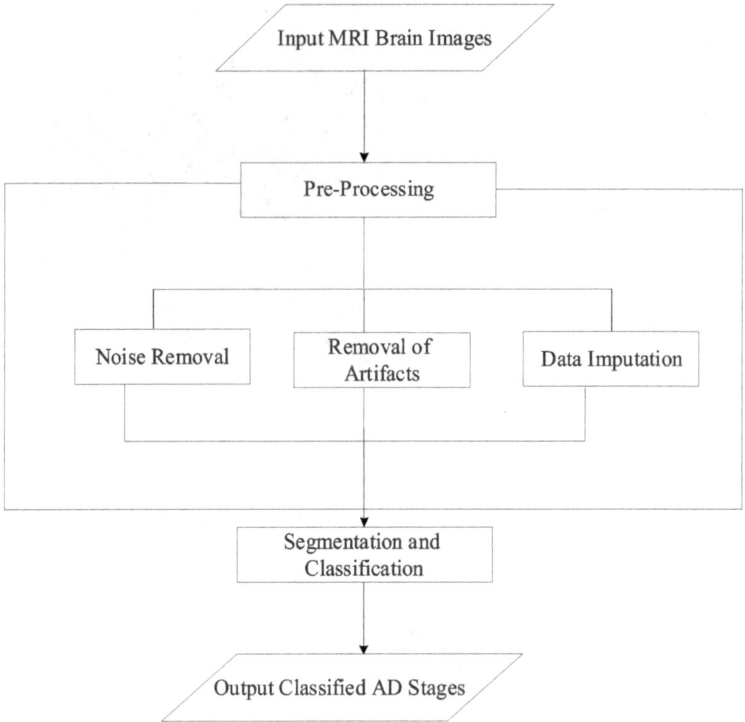

Fig. 3.2 Block Diagram for AD Classification

3.4.1 Progressive Switching Median (PSM) Filter

The median filter is commonly used to suppress noise in an image. It performs better suppression than the mean filter in terms of noise suppression and details preservation. The Median filter provides a filtering rate of 80 % and above. [P.Shanmugavadivu and Eliahim Jeevaraj P.S. 2012]. This order statistic spatial filters' response is based on the computation of the median of the pixels convolved by a kernel and median and placing it in the in-process pixel. The median filters are proved to perform a higher degree of noise suppression, on impulse noise corrupted images.

The progressive switching median filter is designed to handle the images corrupted with impulse noise. It uses two distinct phases, namely, noise detection and noise correction. The first phase constructs a binary matrix as a result of noise detection. In the second phase, through several iterations, noise suppression is implemented. During iterations, both noise detection and filtering processes are repeated that increases the computational time [Boo S T 2009]. The PSM filter observed to preserve the boundary pixels in an image, making it helpful for visual examination and measurement. However, it has the drawback of removing both the noise and the fine details.

3.4.2 Region of Interest (RoI)

The RoI is a built-in procedure of MatLab is most widely used in medical imaging that elicits the boundaries of the RoI or target objects. The RoI can be taken as a polygonal selection from a 2D map in Geographic Information Systems (GIS). The RoI describes the boundaries of an object under investigation. The researchers use this RoI tool to remove the artifacts while extracting the brain region extraction, otherwise known as skull-stripping.

3.4.3 Morphological Operations

Image processing techniques are based on set theory, is mathematical morphology. Typically, morphological operations are used to remove imperfections during segmentation. Most of the image processing operations are designed on mathematical, statistical, and probabilistic principles. Typically, morphological operations are used to process the segmented sub-images using the structuring element. The morphological operations are Dilation, Erosion, Opening, and Closing [Gonzalez, R.C, 2009].

3.4.4 Data Imputation

3.4.4.1 Handling Missing Data

The data imputation of information or a missing value is one of the most important data pre-processing processes. Usually, most medical records are incomplete. The removal of the incomplete instances from the datasets may mislead the interpretation and inferences of datasets. An appropriate imputation technique helps in estimating the missing data. The common imputation types are mean / mode imputation, fuzzy unordered rule induction algorithm based imputation, decision tree imputation, and other machine learning algorithms used to impute the missing values.

Most of the real-life information sets are incomplete its nature. [Zemouri R, 2019]. It is quite common to encounter the problem of missing data while constructing the datasets. The pattern of data imputation is decided based on the nature of the data attributes.

In particular, techniques for handling missing values are either linear such as deletion, assigning the most popular values, arithmetic mean for the numeric attribute or parallel techniques where algorithms for rule induction are used to predict missing values attributes. However, each method has its own merits and demerit, but a few works [Jerez J.M 2010] showed that irrelevant data imputation on information may corrupt data interpretation and mislead the subsequent assessment by introducing bias. Bias is the predicted value from the actual values. If the average predicted values are far from the actual values, then the bias is high. While scientists employ several methods for the imputation of missing value, most of the methods are single imputation methods [Peugh, J.L in 2004]. Deleting cases, imputation of a mean value, maximum probability, and other statistical methods are the most common missing value imputation techniques. In recent years, in several clinical and other incomplete datasets, research has explored machine learning techniques as a method for the imputation of missing values.

A characteristic with numerical data such as a person's age or clinical MR brain image can use it. The mean or modes of the function can be calculated and replaced by the missing values. However, this technique can negate the loss of information, which results in better than removing rows and columns. Replacing the three approximations mentioned above is a statistical approach to managing the missing values, referred to as information leaking.

The general steps involved in data cleaning is shown in Fig. 3.3

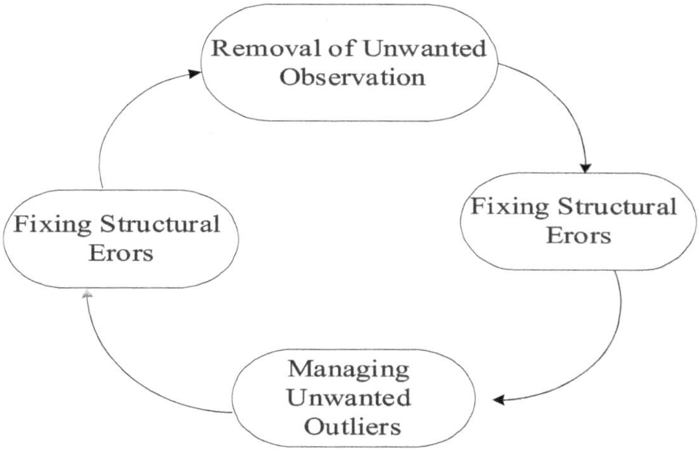

Fig. 3.3 Steps involved in Data Cleaning

3.4.4.2 Removal of unwanted observation

The data cleaning involves the removal of duplicate/redundant or meaningless values. Double observations occur most often in the compilation of information, and irrelevant observations are those that do not effectively match the specific problem one attempts to resolve. The essential aspects of imputation are listed below.

- Redundant observations significantly change the effectiveness as the information repeats and can contribute unfaithfully to the wrong side.
- Any information that does not add any value can be dropped.

3.4.4.3 One-Hot Encoding

One-Hot encoding is the most widespread and commonly used approach, and it works very well unless the categorical variable large in number. This coding creates new (binary) columns, indicating the presence of each possible value from the original data.

MRI ID	Gender	Hand
OASIS _MR_01	M	R
OASIS _MR_02	F	L
OASIS _MR_03	M	R
OASIS _MR_04	F	L

→

MRI ID	Gender	Hand
OASIS _MR_01	0	0
OASIS _MR_02	1	1
OASIS _MR_03	0	0
OASIS _MR_04	1	1

Fig. 3.4 One-Hot Encoding on Categorical Data

The most commonly used coding system is one hot coding. It compares every level to a specified reference point of the categorical variable. The one-hot encoding with 'n' observations and 'd' distinct values converts a single variable into d binary variables, each with n observations. The coding with dichotomous values 0 and 1 are suitably used to code gender and hand, as shown in Fig. 3.4 [Lantz Box, 2013].

3.5 CONCLUSION

The data and image processing techniques for medical diagnosis and AD classification have used the pre-processing component as required. The RoI and morphological operations are used in segmentation methods, and one-hot coding is used for data imputation to estimate the missing values in the clinical dataset.

CHAPTER 4

MR BRAIN IMAGE SEGMENTATION METHODS

4.1 INTRODUCTION

Skull Stripping is an inevitable computer-assisted medical brain image pre-processing mechanism that mainly aims to segregate the non-designated regions and extract the designated brain regions. The resultant brain region images are further subjected to diagnostic analysis to discover brain diseases/ disorders. This chapter presents an efficient image segmentation method named; Threshold and Morphological Operations based Segmentation (TMOS) for skull stripping, exclusively designed for MRI brain images. It has two phases; the first phase localizes the brain region using Region of Interest (RoI), and the second phase, morphological operations are applied to precisely extract the brain region by stripping out the skull. The performance of TMOS is validated using the Minimal Interval Resonance Image in Alzheimer's Disease (MIRIAD) dataset [Malone 2013]. The efficiency of the proposed TMOS method is confirmed through the visual perception of the segmented regions.

The fully/semi-automated brain image analysis aims to discover brain abnormalities/ disorders and other diagnoses. Skull stripping is an essential step in extracting the brain regions for morphometric studies of Magnetic Resonance Images (MRI). This demand and requirement justify the development of TMOS.

TMOS is designed using Region of Interest (RoI) and morphological operations. The primary objective of TMOS is to accurately segment the brain image, with minimum computational and time complexity. It is apparent to underline that TMOS combats the common bottlenecks of segmentation algorithm terms, namely Threshold and Morphological Operations based Segmentation. Hence, TMOS is confirmed to be an ideal pre-processing tool in brain image processing and analysis. The flow diagram of the TMOS is depicted in Fig. 4.1.

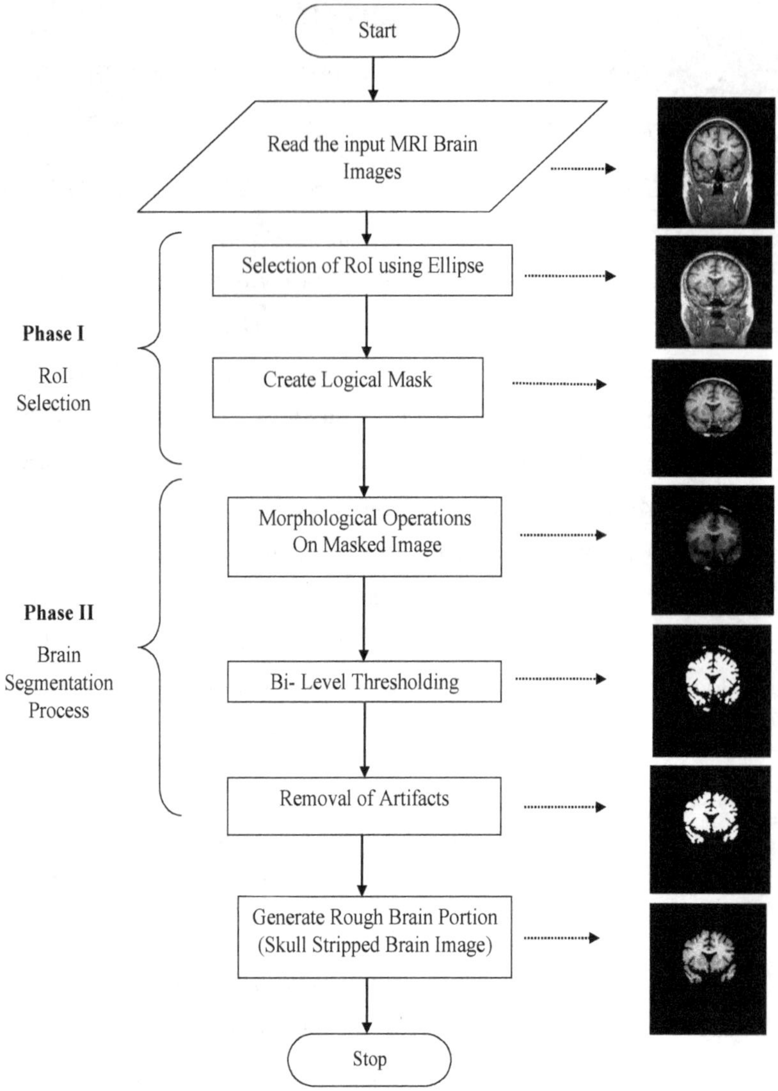

Fig. 4.1 Flowchart of TMOS

The following sections described the methodology of TMOS and the analysis of its results. The MRI brain segmentation using TMOS involves RoI, thresholding-based region selection, and morphological operations based segmentation.

In TMOS, the input MRI is binarized using Otsu's thresholding *[Otsu.N. 1979]* wherein the selection of threshold is automatically made using *[Liao P.S.2001]* to proven global thresholding method which iterates through all the possible threshold values to separate the foreground from the background optimally. The process of brain segmentation is optimized with the automatic/semi-automatic selection of RoI. In TMOS, the RoI is chosen based on the elliptical mask using an interactive tool is Matlab R2013A.

The masking operations concerning the chosen RoI facilitate the selection of pixels is confined within the boundary of RoI. The pixels bounded by the RoI are preserved while the remaining pixels are discarded using the *ellipse* convolution filter. This convolution operation enables us to separate the RoI from the MRI image, leaving out the remaining pixels (i.e.) unwanted pixels. In general, the morphological image operators viz., *erosion, dilation, opening*, and *closing* are applied on digital images separately or in combination, to refine the process of segmentation using structuring elements of varying sizes, as required. The TMOS uses *opening* and *closing* operations for the brain's skull stripping and RoI selection. The *opening* of A by B is succeeded by *dilation*. The *opening* of A by B is:

$$A \circ B = (A \ominus B) \oplus B \tag{4.1}$$

The morphological *closing* is similar to *dilation* in which the boundaries of the foreground regions are based on the given structuring element. The *closing* of A by B is:

$$A \bullet B = (A \ominus B) \ominus B \tag{4.2}$$

The TMOS algorithm is given in Algorithm 4.1

4.1 Algorithmic Description for TMOS

Input: Grayscale Image I (Normal/AD)

Output: Extracted Brain Portion

Begin

Step 1: Read the input MR brain images

Step 2: Select the coordinates for RoI selection with ellipse

Step 3: Set color draw RoI boundary

Step 4: Add a new position call back to RoI object

Step 5: Adjust and limit the ellipse boundary using X and Y limit

Step 6**:** Create Logical mask in the image

Step 7: Define Structuring Element (SE) and apply erosion

Step 8: With Structure information, apply dilation

Step 9: Apply Top-Hat filtering for refinement

Step 10: Apply morphological operations to separate the brain images using the Opening and Closing function

Step 11: Segment brain image using Otsu's threshold method

Step 12: Convert the segmented image into a binary image

Step 13: Remove artifacts in the binary image

Step 14: Segment the brain image

End

4.2 RESULTS AND DISCUSSION

The visual perception of the segmented results validates the effectiveness of TMOS. The indicative results of TMOS for Normal Control and AD affected brain images are given in Fig. 4.2 & Fig. 4.3 respectively. TMOS is implemented using Matlab R2013A.

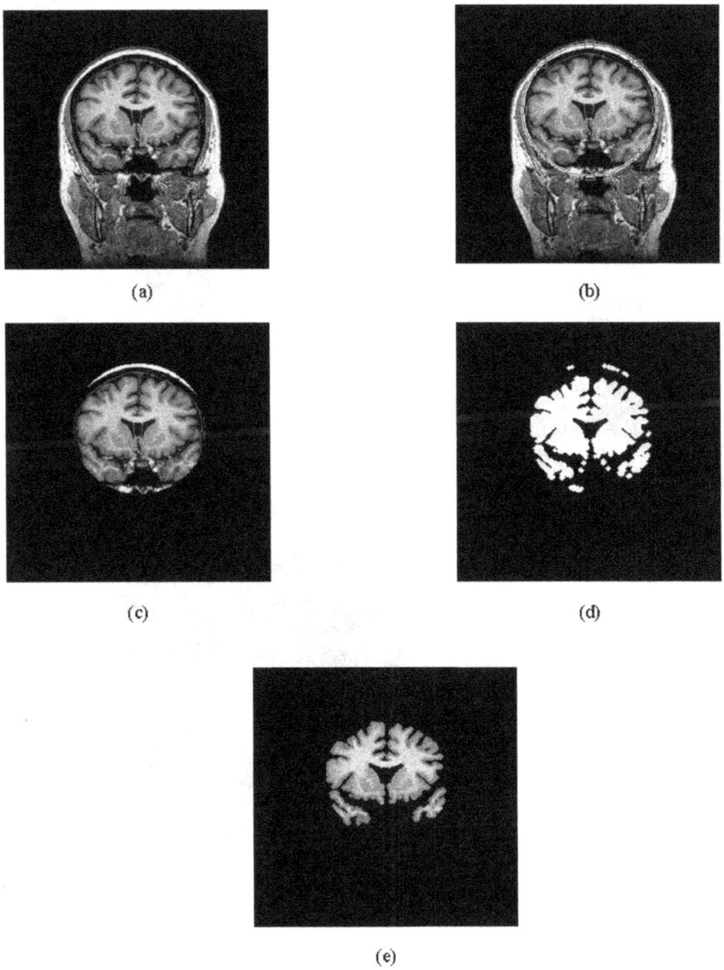

Fig. 4.2 Skull - Stripped Normal MRI Brain image; (a) Original Image (b) RoI Mask (c) Region of Interest (d) Opening and Closing of Morphological Operation (e) Extracted Brain Image

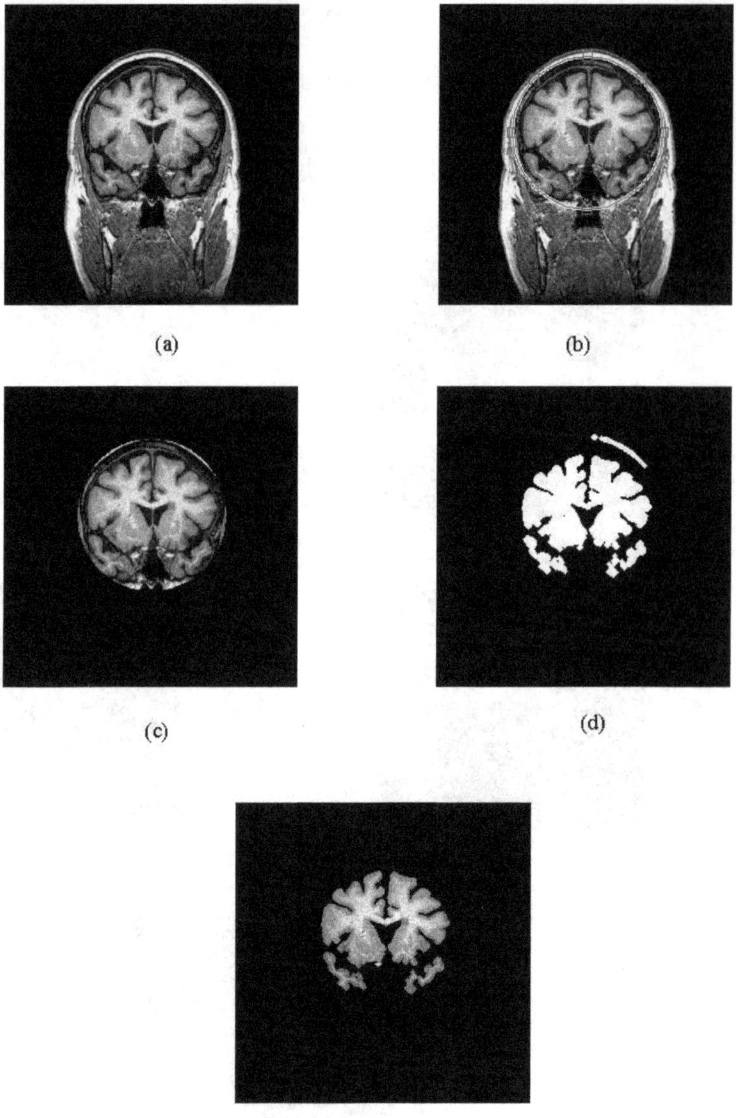

(e)

Fig. 4.3 Skull - Stripped AD MRI Brain image; (a) Original Image (b) RoI Mask (c) Region of Interest (d) Opening and Closing of Morphological Operation (e) Extracted Brain Image

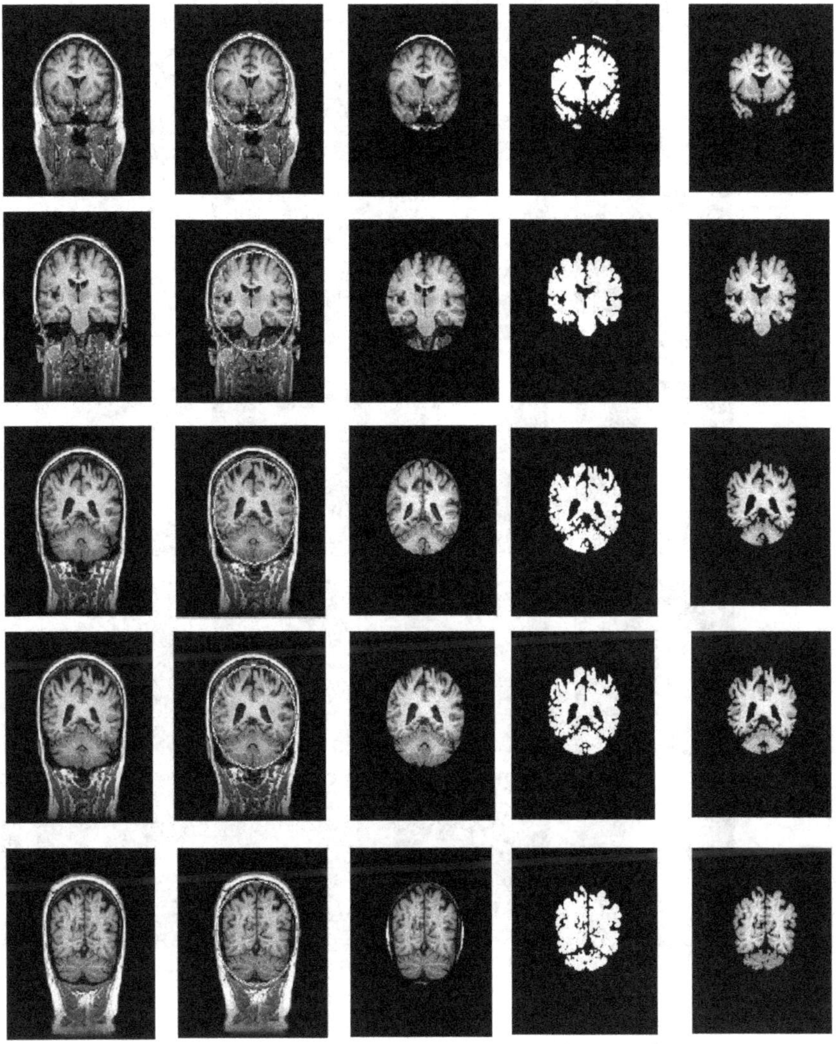

(a) (b) (c) (d) (e)

Fig. 4.4 Skull Stripped Brain Images; (a) Normal MR Brain Image (b) Selection of RoI Mask (c) Detection of RoI (d) Artifacts Removed Brain Images (e) Segmented Brain Images by TMOS (Skull Stripped)

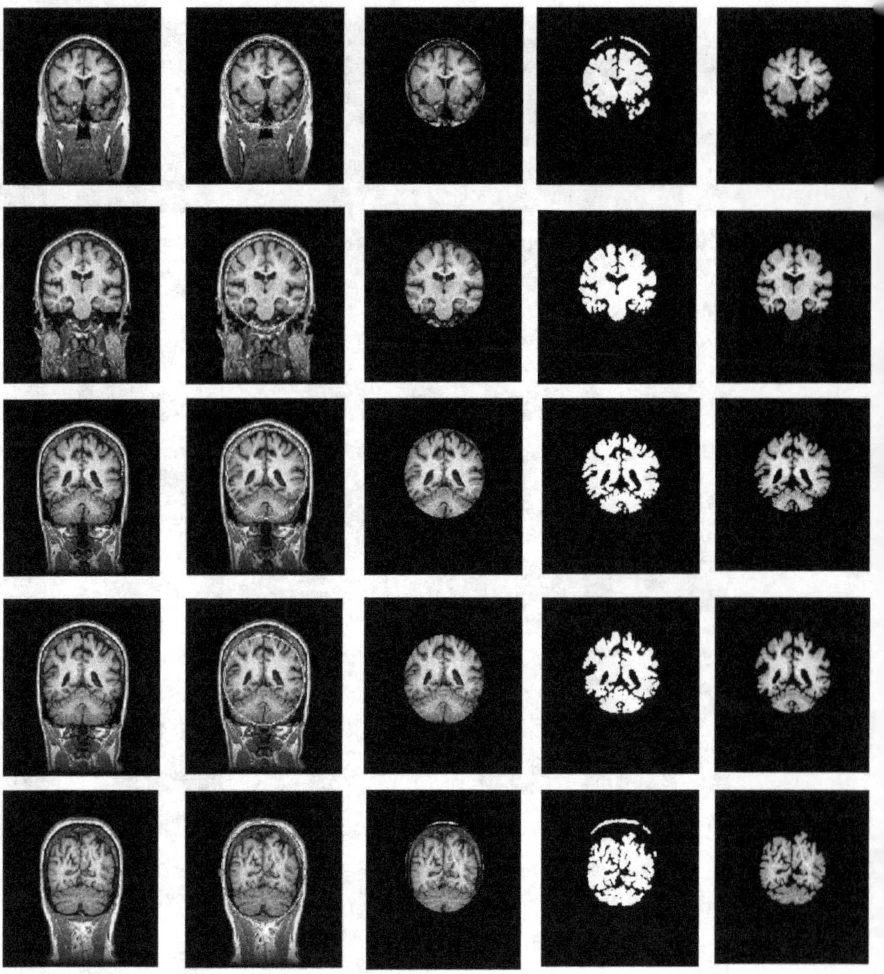

(a) (b) (c) (d) (e)

Fig. 4.5 Skull Stripped Brain Image (a) AD-affected MR Brain Image (b) Selection of RoI Mask (c) Detection of RoI (d) Artifacts Removed Brain Images (e) Segmented Brain Images by TMOS (Skull Stripped)

The sample images from the dataset and their corresponding segmented images are depicted in Fig. 4.3 and Fig. 4.4. In Fig. 4.3(a) and Fig. 4.5, a sample Normal brain images from the MIRIAD dataset is shown, whereas in Fig. 4.3 (b), the output of TMOS on (a) are given likewise the AD sample AD affected images are given in, and the respective results are given in Fig. 4.4 (b)

4.3 MR BRAIN IMAGE SEGMENTATION USING K-MEANS AND CLUSTERING AND EXPECTATION MAXIMIZATION (MRB-kM-EM)

The research work on segmentation uses k-Means Clustering and Expectation Maximization (MRB-KM-EM) that performs skull-stripping, impulse noise removal, segmentation of brain tissues, and classification of brain images. The method titled, MRB-KM-EM employs morphology bound segmentation for skull removal, Progressive Switching Median Filter (PSMF) for noise suppression in the input brain images. The brain tissues are segmented into white matter and gray matter using k-means clustering and expectation maximization. The outcomes of this research can be used to analyze the brain features and detect AD's presence/ absence.

4.3.1 Methodology of MRB-kM-EM

The computational mechanisms of MRB-km-EM its components are: (a) Contour Based Brain Segmentation for skull stripping (CBS); (b) Progressive Switching Median Filter (PSM) for noise suppression; and (c) Brain Segmentation using k-Means Clustering and Expectation Maximization. The flowchart is shown in Fig. 4.8. dedicates the control flow of MRB-kM-EM.

A. Skull Stripping in Brain Images

The foremost task in MR brain image segmentation is skull stripping that aims to remove non-brain regions *[Church J.C. 2008]*. ADD–kM-EM uses Contour Based Brain Segmentation (CBS) method to remove the skull regions from normal and AD-affected MR brain images *[Sun. T., 1994]*.

B. ***Noise Suppression***

The Progressive Switching Median Filter (PSM) is a median-based filter used to remove the impulse noise from highly corrupted images *[Wang.Z. 1999]*. It is applied to the skull-stripped images to adaptively suppress the noise on the corrupted pixels, preserving the uncorrupted pixels intact. The PSM estimates the intensity of the corrupted in the given image.

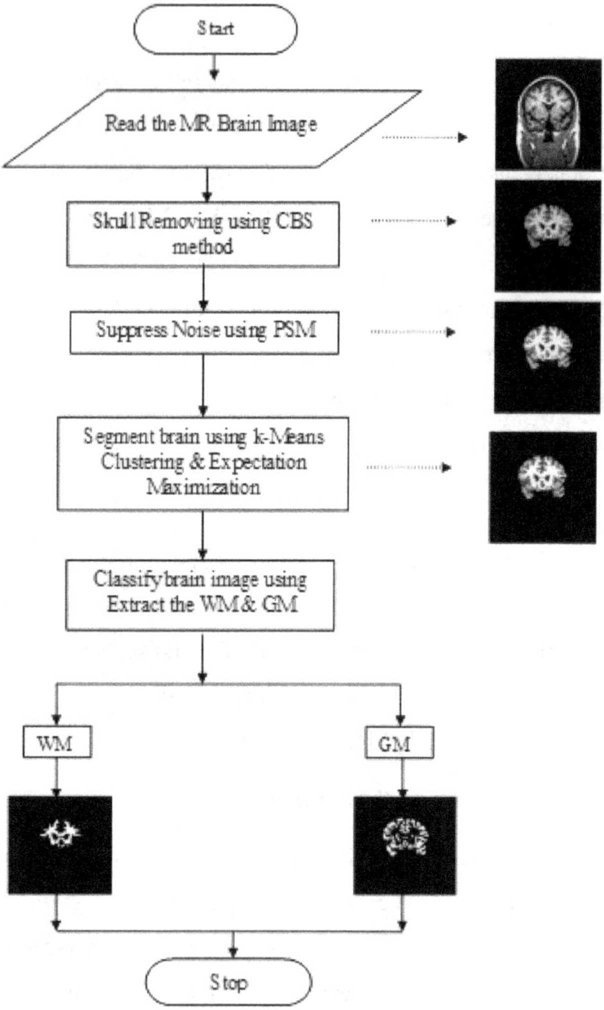

Fig. 4.6 Flowchart of MRB-kM-EM

C. Brain Segmentation

4.2 Algorithmic Description of MRB-kM-EM

Input: *k (Number of Clusters) and Brain Image Dataset (with n objects).*

Output: *A set of k-clusters*

begin

1. Randomly select *k* objects as the initial cluster centers.
2. Assign each object to a cluster with which the object is the most similar, using the objects' mean in the cluster.
3. Compute: *Mean* of clusters.
4. If the current *mean* is not equal to the previous *mean,* go to Step 2.
5. Output the clusters.

End

Expectation-Maximization (EM) algorithm is an iterative method to compute maximum probability or Maximum A Posterior (MAP) computation of statistical models, wherein the model depends on the overlooked latent parameters. The EM iteration toggles between Expectation (E) and Maximization (M). The Expectation function estimates the expected log-likelihood of the parameters, and the maximization (M) step maximizes the expected log-likelihood. Despite the k-Means algorithm being simple to compute, it suffers due to getting stuck in local optima. This method has the mechanism of assigning data points partially to multiple clusters, instead of assigning it to a single cluster. The probability distribution controls the task of partial assignment.

4.3 Algorithmic Description of Expectation Maximization

Input: *Cluster number k, Image Database, Stopping criteria.*

Output: *A set of k-clusters with a weight that maximizes log-likelihood function.*

begin

1. *Expectation (E):* For each database record x, compute the membership probability of x in each cluster $h = 1, \ldots, k$.
2. *Maximization (M):* Update the probability weight of parameters.
3. *Stopping Criteria:* ***If*** stopping criteria are satisfied to stop,

   Else

   Set $j = j + 1$ and go to (1).

End

The overall procedural description of the MRB-kM-EM is given below.

4.4 Algorithmic Description of MRB-kM-EM (Proposed)

begin

Step 1: Start.

Step 2: Read the input brain images.

Step 3: Remove the Skull in input brain images using the CBS method.

Step 4: Noise Suppression using PSM filters.

Step 5: Segment using k-Means clustering and EM method.

Step 6: Stop.

End

4.4 RESULTS AND DISCUSSION

The MRB-kM-BM is tested on the 850 brain images of IBSR and MIRIAD databases for brain image segmentation, and the results are recorded for human visual perception. The sample images of the processed datasets of IBSR and MIRIAD are shown in Fig. 4.7, 4.8 and 4.9 respectively. In these images, the input images are given in (a); skull stripped images, and PSM filtered images of (a) are shown in (b) & (c); the outcome of MRB-kM-EM are subsequently clustered, WM and GM are given in (d), (e) and (f) respectively.

Table 4.1 Similarity Measures of MRB-kM-EM (Proposed)

Similarity Measures				
Images	**JACCARD**		**DICE**	
	WM	**GM**	**WM**	**GM**
1_brainslice_20	0.7447	0.5696	0.8424	0.7086
1_brainslice_24	0.8217	0.8122	0.9021	0.8964
1_brainslice_25	0.8969	0.8451	0.9456	0.9160
2_brainslice_28	0.8921	0.8301	0.9430	0.9072
3_brainslice_29	0.9168	0.8858	0.9566	0.9394
4_brainslice_13	0.9821	0.9352	0.9215	0.9075
Average	**0.875717**	**0.813**	**0.918533**	**0.879183**

In the MRB-kM-EM method, the lowest segmented value of 0.5696 for GM was produced and has shown the accuracy of 91% better result of WM on our selected dataset. The results obtained for this method in terms of Jaccard and Dice confirm the similar measure for WM and GM are 87% and 81%, respectively. Likewise, it is 91% and 87% from Dice.

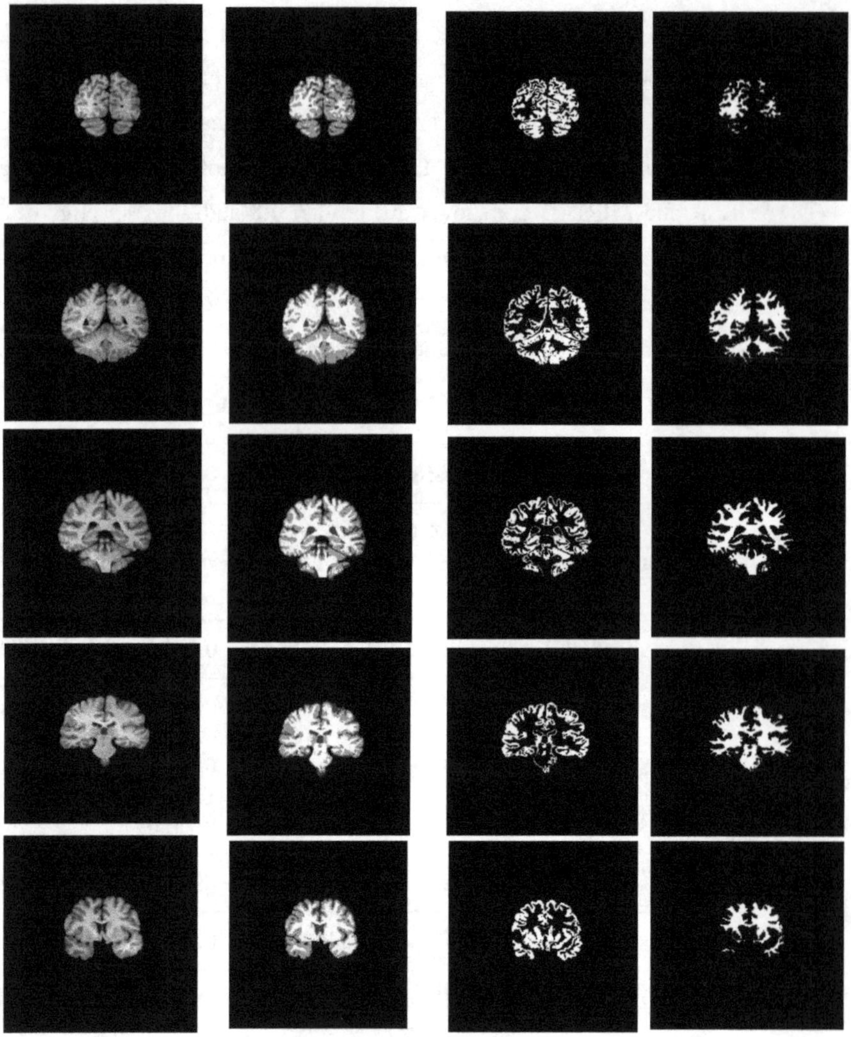

(a) (b) (c) (d)

Fig. 4.7 Results of MRB-kM-EM on Normal Brain Image (IBSR) (a) Input Images (b) MRB-KM-EM Cluster (c) WM (d) GM

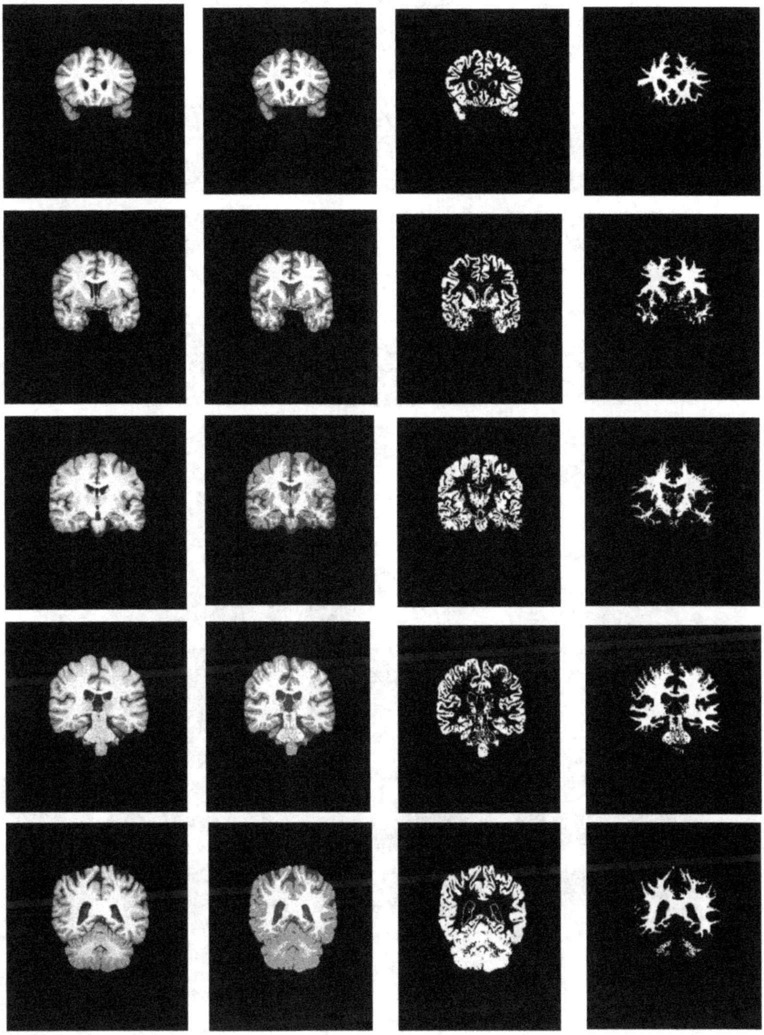

(a) (b) (c) (d)

Fig. 4.8 Results of MRB-kM-EM on Normal Brain Image (MIRIAD) (a) Input Images (b) MRB-kM-EM Cluster (c) WM (d) GM

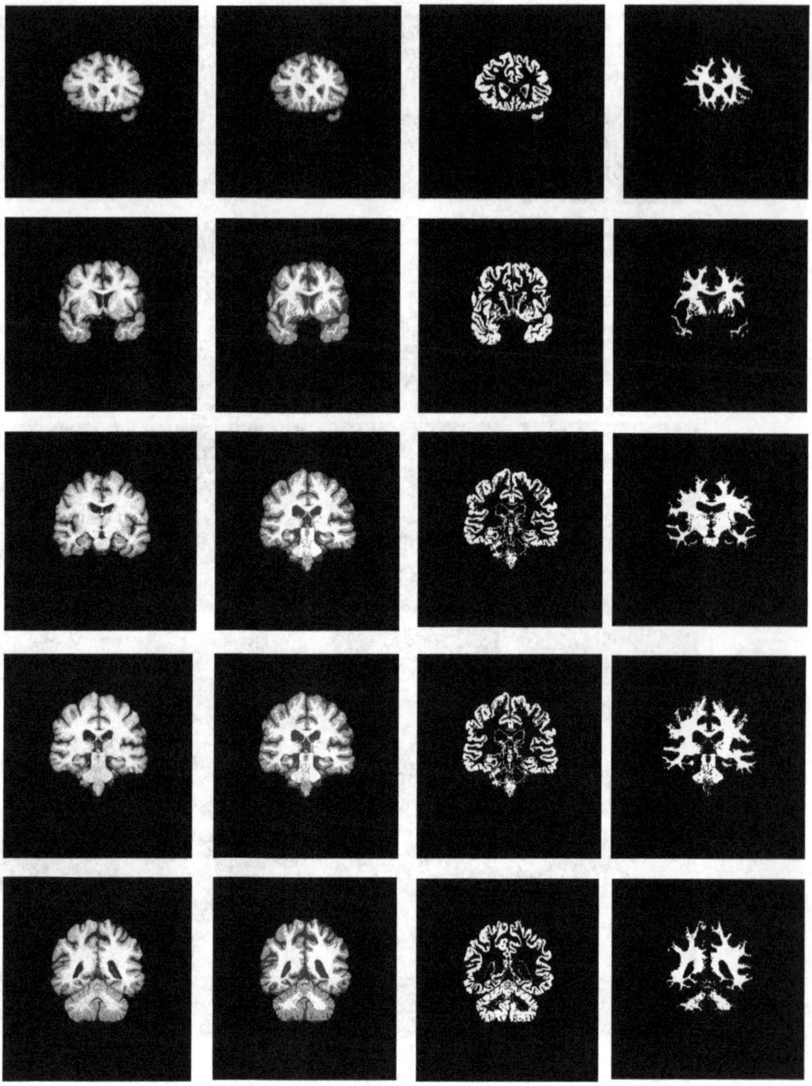

(a) (b) (c) (d)

Fig. 4.9 Results of MRB-kM-EM on AD Brain Image (MIRIAD)
(a) Input Images (b) MRB-kM-EM Cluster (c) WM (d) GM

The proposed MRB-kM-EM exhibits a high accuracy in segmenting the brain region/issues accurately into the White matter and Gray matter. The visual perception of the segmented.

4.5 CONCLUSION

In this chapter, two segmentation methods, TMOS, and kM-EM. The results of this research work directly find a place in the detection of WM and GM.

A new technique called TMOS for brain portion extraction is discussed in this chapter. It is designed using RoI selection and morphological operations for skull stripping. The developed method was tested on T1-weighted MRI brain images of MIRIAD (Minimal Interval Resonance Imaging in Alzheimer Disease) dataset. The visual inception of the skull stripped brain confirms the efficiency of the proposed TMOS. Due to its accuracy, this method finds several applications, and it is apparent that the devised TMOS accurately segments the brain regions from MRI brain images of two different datasets. The results of the TMOS can be directly used for a higher degree of image processing.

A robust and straightforward MR brain segmentation method, MRB-kM-EM for normal and abnormal brain images, is proposed. This method is successful in segmenting the brain tissues using the kM-EM method. The automatic segmentation of WM, GM, and CSF can be used to quantify neurological damage in brain images, especially in AD detection.

CHAPTER 5

MULTINOMIAL LOGISTIC REGRESSION MODEL FOR CLASSIFICATION OF ALZHEIMER'S DISEASE

5.1 INTRODUCTION

Alzheimer's disease (AD) is a neuro-disorder that impedes the physical, mental functions and abilities of aged persons, while the cognitive functions deteriorate and eventually lead to death [NIH USA 2013]. Early analysis of AD is widely sought for the development of new treatment strategies. This chapter presents a classification technique based on the principle Multinomial Logistic Regression Classifier model to detect the stages of AD. The diagnosis of AD images is made using feature representations for classification using similar brain patterns and pixel intensities. Machine Learning techniques can learn such MRI delay, MRI ID, sex, hand, visit, etTIV, nWBV, CDR, MMSE, and group representation from the data. This multi-classifier model can handle the classes, namely Healthy Control (HC) and Mild AD, Very Mild AD, and Moderate AD. Experiments are performed using the Open Access Series of Imaging Studies (OASIS) dataset and to validate the multi-class classification AD. This model's performance was validated concerning the precision, recall, and F1-score on the validation set.

Full or semi-automated brain image analysis aims to discover brain abnormalities/ disorders and other diagnoses. Early detection and classification of AD are needed to provide necessary treatments to the patients at an early stage. Magnetic Resonance Imaging (MRI) is a diagnostic tool that gives high-resolution images and high contrast for the brain's gray and white matter. In particular, the prediction capabilities of machine learning methods are ideal for many clinical applications. One area of Neuroimaging research where these techniques have gained attention is in the early detection and diagnosis of Alzheimer's disease (AD).

Machine learning classification techniques have been explored for improving technology using Big Data and Artificial Intelligence. This chapter proposes a new prediction scheme for MRI clinical data called Alzheimer's disease analysis using a Multinomial Logistic Regression Classifier (AD-MNLR). The proposed model is trained to detect the early stages of AD.

5.2 METHODOLOGY OF AD-MNLR

5.2.1 AD - Multinomial Logistic Regression Classifier (AD-MNLR)

Logistic Regression is a statistical method for predicting binary classes. The outcome or target variables are dichotomous. Dichotomous is the one that has only two possible classes for solving the binary classification problem. Another category of classification is multinomial classification, where multiple class values are present in the target dataset.

In this chapter, a general framework for the analysis and prediction of AD, based on the multinomial logistic regression model, using a multi-class classifier model is proposed.

They are two types of terms describing the logistic regression models:

A. **Binary Logistic Regression**: The target variable only predicts "Yes" or "No".

B. **Multinomial Logistic Regression**: The target variables can predict “Multi-Classes”.

5.2.2 Multinomial Logistic Regression (MNLR)

Multinomial Logistic Regression is used more frequently than discriminant function analysis because it does not have assumptions [Valencia, N 2018]. Multinomial Logistic Regression does have assumptions, such as the assumption of independence among the dependent variable choices. This assumption states that membership in one category is not related to the choice of membership of another category (i.e., the dependent variable). The assumption of independence can be tested with the Hausman-McFadden test. Furthermore, multinomial logistic Regression also assumes non-perfect separation.

There are different parameter estimation techniques based on the inferential goals of multinomial logistic regression analysis.

This method uses multinomial logistic Regression with an L2 penalty on a subset of clinical data classification. It uses the 'newton-cg' algorithm for hyper-parameter fine-tuning. The computational steps of the AD-MNLR are listed in Algorithm 5.1, and its flow diagram is presented in Fig. 5.1.

Hyperparameters Used in The Model:

1. **Penalty: (data type: L2)**

   It is used to specify the norm built in the penalization.

2. **Dual: (data type: boolean; data value: 0 or 1)**

   The dual formulation is only implemented for the L2 penalty with liblinear solver.

3. **Fit_intercept :(data type: bool; data value: True)**

   Specifies if a constant (bias or intercept) should be added to the decision function.

4. **Intercept_scaling: (data type: float; data value:1)**

   In this case, x becomes [x, self intercept_scalling], the synthetic features with a constant value equal to intercept_scalling is appended to the instance vector. The intercept becomes.

   $$intercept_{scaling} * synthetic\_feature\_Weight$$

5. **Class_weight: (data type: balanced; data value: 30)**

   The balanced mode uses the value of y to automatically adjust weights inversely proportional to class frequencies in the input data.

6. **random _state: (data type: *integer;* data value: 50)**

   the seed of the pseudo-random number generator to use when shuttling the data if int.

7. **Solver: (data algorithm: newton-cg)**

   The algorithm is used for the optimization problem.

   It is used for the multinomial problems and handles multinomial loss schemes.

8. **Multi_class: (data type: *integer;* data value: multinomial)**

   For multinomial, the loss is minimized to fit across the entire probability distribution.

5.1 Algorithmic Description of AD-MNLR

Input: Clinical Data from MRI Brain Images

Output: Classification of Alzheimer's Disease Stages

begin

Phase – I: Pre-Processing

Step 1: Read the clinical data

Step 2: Data imputation for filling in missing values.

Step 3: One-Hot Encoding of categorical input data

Step 4: Split data for training and testing.

Phase – II: Classification

Step 5: Train the data using a Multinomial Logistic Regression model

Step 6: Tuning the MNLR classifier hyperparameters using newton-cg Algorithm

Step 7: Train the MNLR model

Step 8: Test the model on validation data.

Step 9: Performance Evaluation & Results

end

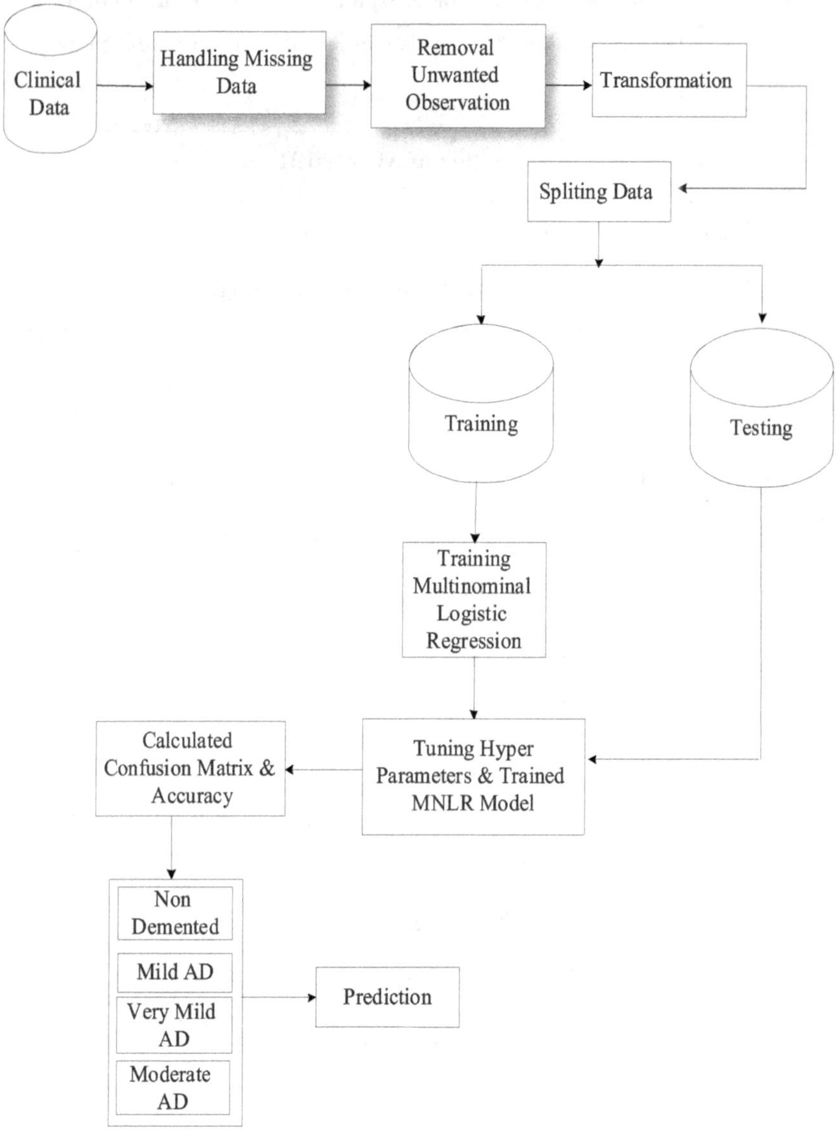

Fig. 5.1 Block Diagram for AD-MNLR

For comparative analysis, the results of Alzheimer's disease classification are also recorded. The classification is done by using the AD-MNLR model.

5.3 RESULTS AND DISCUSSION

OASIS clinical data has been used to analyze the performance of the proposed model. The data is divided into four classes; Mild AD, Moderate AD, Non-Demented and Very Mild AD. The performance for each of the available classes has been recorded to identify the proposed model's efficiency in detecting the various stages of Alzheimer's Disease. The training data has been pre-processed, transformed, and passed to the AD-MNLR model. The model has been implemented using Python and scikit library. The results obtained using the AD-MNLR model have been recorded at various stages. Improvement in the performance after each pre-processing stage has been analyzed. Results are compared in terms of Precision, Accuracy, Recall, F1-Score, and Support.

Table 5.1 Performance of OASIS Clinical Data with missing values

Group	Precision	Recall	F1-Score	Support
Mild AD	0.00	0.00	0.00	15
Moderate AD	0.00	0.00	0.00	0
Non-Demented	0.51	0.58	0.55	62
Very Mild AD	0.24	0.23	0.23	35
Classification Report				
Macro Avg	0.19	0.20	0.19	112
Weighted Avg	0.36	0.39	0.37	112
Accuracy: 0.39285714285714285 (39.28%)				

The classification performance of MNLR is depicted in Table 5.1 and Fig. 5.2, for precision, recall, and F1-Score. It could be observed that the proposed model exhibits low values of Precision, Recall, F1-Score, and Support in classifying Mild and Moderate AD. The OASIS dataset with 448 data, out of which 112 data are Mild AD; 112 data are Moderate AD; 112 data are Non-demented, and 112 data are Very Mild AD- affected cases. The performance is shown in Fig. 5.3. A support value of zero for Moderate AD indicates the poor-performance nature of the model. It is apparent that the classification accuracy of AD-MNLR is not promising, and the testing accuracy is also quite low.

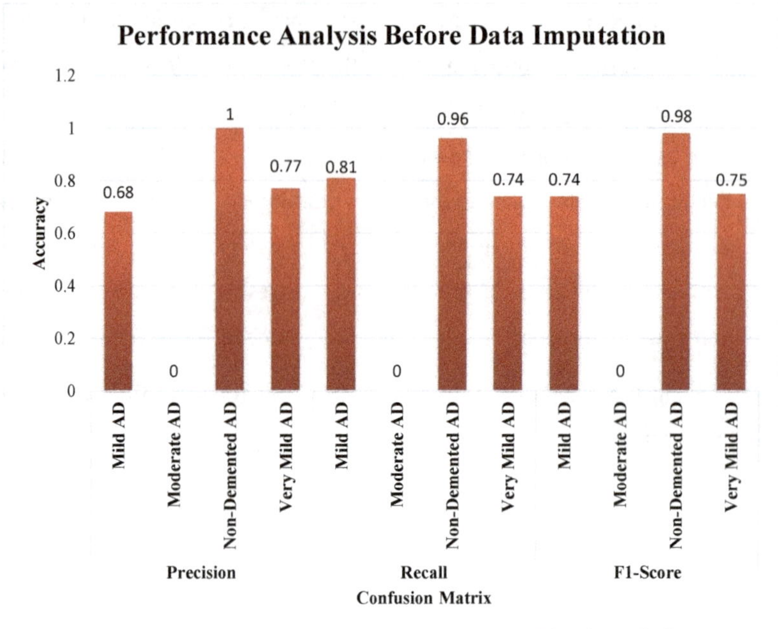

Fig. 5.2 Performance Analysis of OASIS Clinical Data with Missing Values

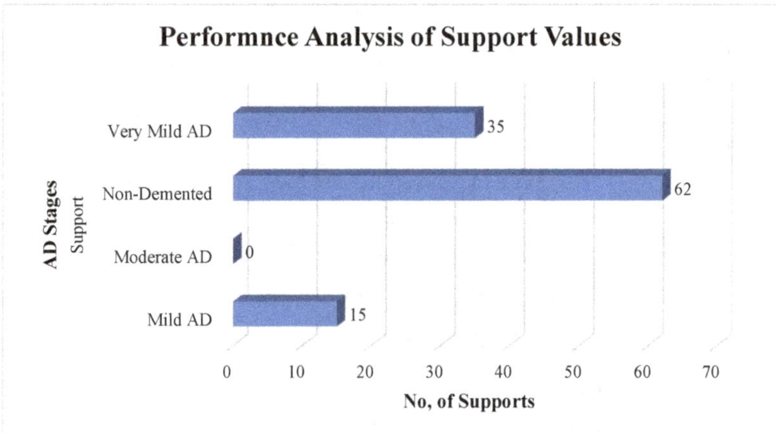

Fig. 5.3 Performance Analysis of Support Values for Missing Data

Data imputation has been applied to the OASIS data and, Table 5.2 and Fig. 5.4 show the results after applying data imputation using the AD-MNLR model. A slight improvement in the performance could be observed after data imputation. Prediction metrics for Non-Demented and Very Mild AD increased approximately to ~8%. The model performance values for the chosen metrics and the model accuracy were 45.53%, with an increased 6% performance. The Support values recorded for this model also confirm improved performance.

Table 5.2 Performance Analysis of OASIS Clinical Data after Data Imputation

Group	Precision	Recall	F1-Score	Support
Mild AD	0.00	0.00	0.00	14
Moderate AD	0.00	0.00	0.00	14
Non-Demented	0.59	0.57	0.58	65
Very Mild AD	0.35	0.42	0.38	33
Classification Report				
Macro Avg	0.31	0.33	0.32	112
Weighted Avg	0.44	0.46	0.45	112
Accuracy: 0.45535714285714285 (45.53%)				

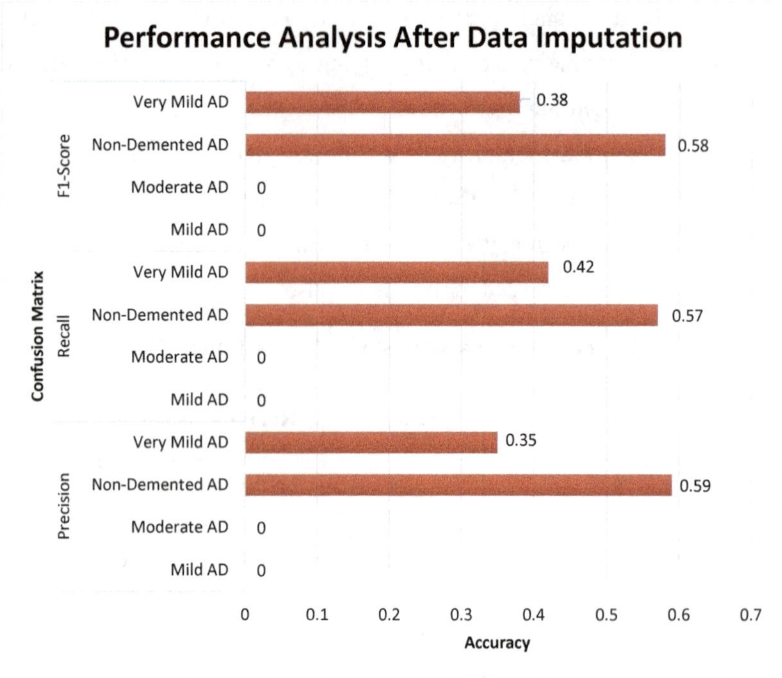

Fig. 5.4 Performance Analysis of OASIS Clinical Data after Data Imputation

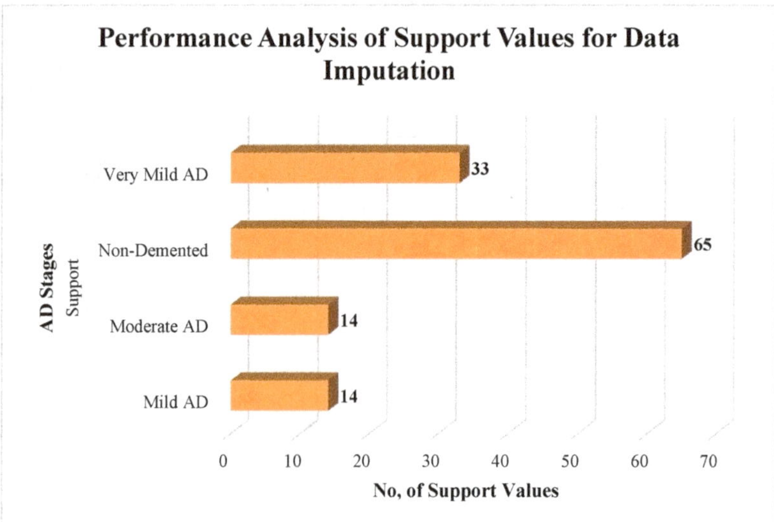

Fig. 5.5 Performance Analysis of Support Values after Data Imputation

Table 5.3 Performance analysis of AD-MNLR Model with Hyperparameter Tuning

Group	Precision	Recall	F1-Score	Support
Mild AD	0.68	0.81	0.74	16
Moderate AD	0.00	0.00	0.00	1
Non-Demented	1.00	0.96	0.98	69
Very Mild AD	0.77	0.74	0.75	27
Classification Report				
Macro Avg	0.61	0.63	0.62	112
Weighted Avg	0.90	0.88	0.89	112
Accuracy: 0.8839285714285714 (88.39%)				

The performance analysis after applying all the initial performance enhancement modules are shown in Table 5.3 and Fig. 5.6. A considerable increase in the performance of the model in terms of all the evaluated metrics can be observed. The model's accuracy is observed as 88.39%, and a 43% increase could be observed in the final predictions. Very high performance could be observed in detecting the Non-Demented class, while an acceptable increase of 43%-68% could be observed in precision. Similar increase levels could be observed in terms of all the metrics.

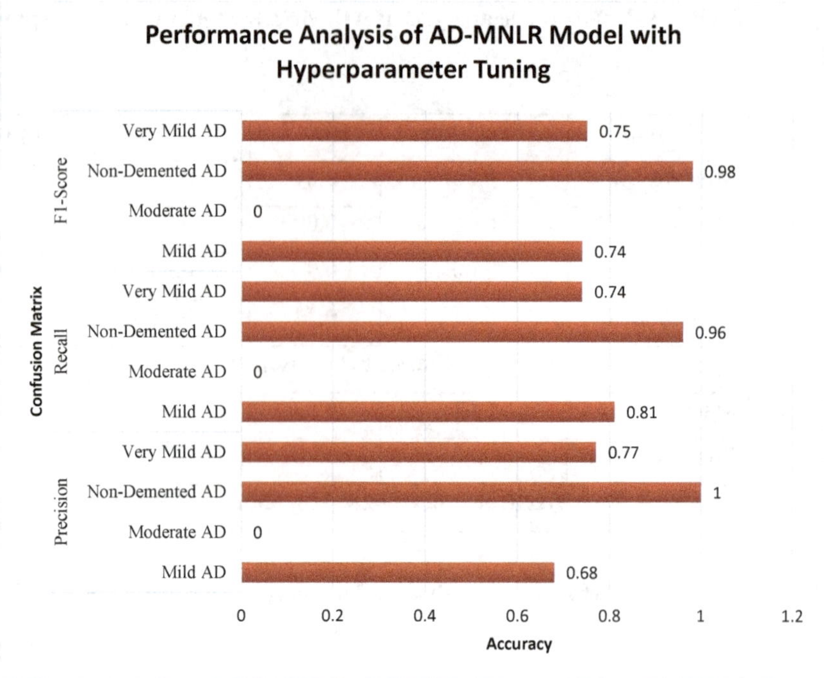

Fig. 5.6 Performance analysis of OASIS Clinical Data for AD-MNLR -HPT Model with Hyperparameter Tuning

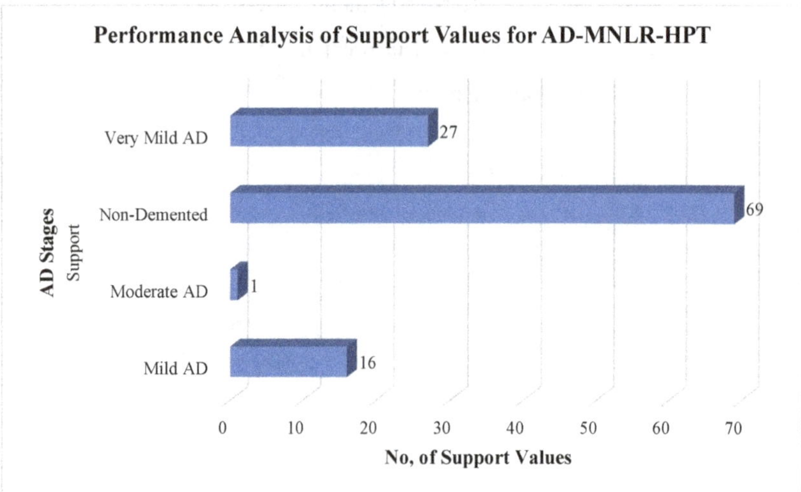

Fig. 5.7 Performance Analysis of Support values for AD-MNLR-HPT Model with Hyperparameter Tuning

Training and test data performance of AD-MNLR-HPT (Hyper Parameter Tuning) is shown in Fig. 5.8. A training accuracy of 0.93 and a test accuracy of 0.88 could be observed. The results indicate that the model has not been over-trained or under-trained. Effective training automatically indicates high performance, which can be observed in the proposed model.

Table 5.4 Comparative Analysis of Training and Testing Accuracy

Method	Training Accuracy	Testing Accuracy
Missing Data	0.74	39.28%
Data Imputation	0.85	45.53%
Tuning Hyperparameters	0.93	88.39%

The comparison of performance after each stage of processing is shown in Table 5.4 and Fig.5.8. It is observed that every stage contributes to substantial improvement in the performance.

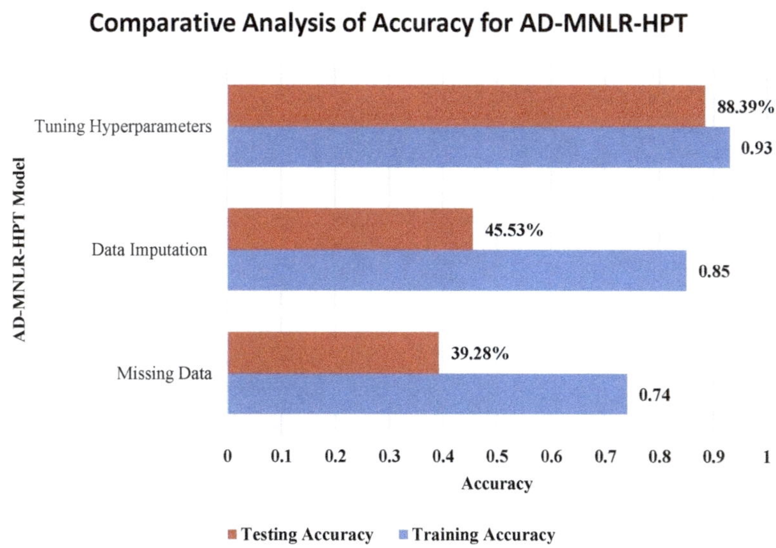

Fig. 5.8 Comparative Analysis of Accuracy for AD-MNLR-HPT

5.4 CONCLUSION

This chapter reports on a Multinomial Logistic Regression to classify Alzheimer's disease from an MRI brain at an early stage using MRI brain analysis. The proposed work brings out and highlights the merits of modified multinomial logistic Regression, in comparison with improved multinomial logistic regression classification method. Hence this approach helps detect AD from the clinical data more precisely and can be used for developing an interactive expert system for early detection of Alzheimer's disease.

This classification method can be divided into two main phases: data-cleaning and classification. The pre-processing includes data imputation method, which utilizes the mode function. Classification is done using the Multinomial Logistic Regression Model. This algorithm can help with the early diagnosis of the stages of AD.

The results of AD-MNLR-HPT serve as a feeder for the newly developed classification techniques described in the next chapter.

CHAPTER 6

ENHANCED TREE BASED CLASSIFIER FOR EFFECTIVE CLASSIFICATION ALZHEIMER'S DISEASE

6.1 INTRODUCTION

Early diagnosis of AD is critical for proper treatment. Machine learning is an artificial intelligence branch that uses various probabilistic methods and optimization to detect Post-Concussion Syndrome (PCS) from large, multipart datasets. This objective has motivated many scientists to concentrate on early Alzheimer's Disease machine learning. The performance of machine learning-based methods for AD classification depends on various factors such as training data, pre-processing, feature selection, and classifiers. This method can cover pre-processing, attributes selection, and classification using association rules. A successful diagnostic solution for AD is provided in the proposed model.

Alzheimer's disease (AD) is a progressive degeneration of brain functions, leading to behavioral and physical dysfunctions, in particular, among the elderly," says the United States National Institutes of Health – National Institute on Aging (NIH-NIA). AD assumes the third place among common disabilities across the world, next to cardiovascular diseases and cancer. AD is also recorded as the sixth major cause of mortality in the USA [Tejada-V.B 2013]. The development of neurodegenerative diseases cannot be detected directly by the visual analysis of radiologists. Neuroimaging is a vital tool in the early diagnosis of neurodegenerative diseases by deriving objective pattern and structural relations from Magnetic Resonance (MR) images.

6.2 DESCRIPTION OF CLASSIFIERS

Classifiers are models that allocate appropriate class labels (from a set of known class labels) to test samples represented as feature vectors.

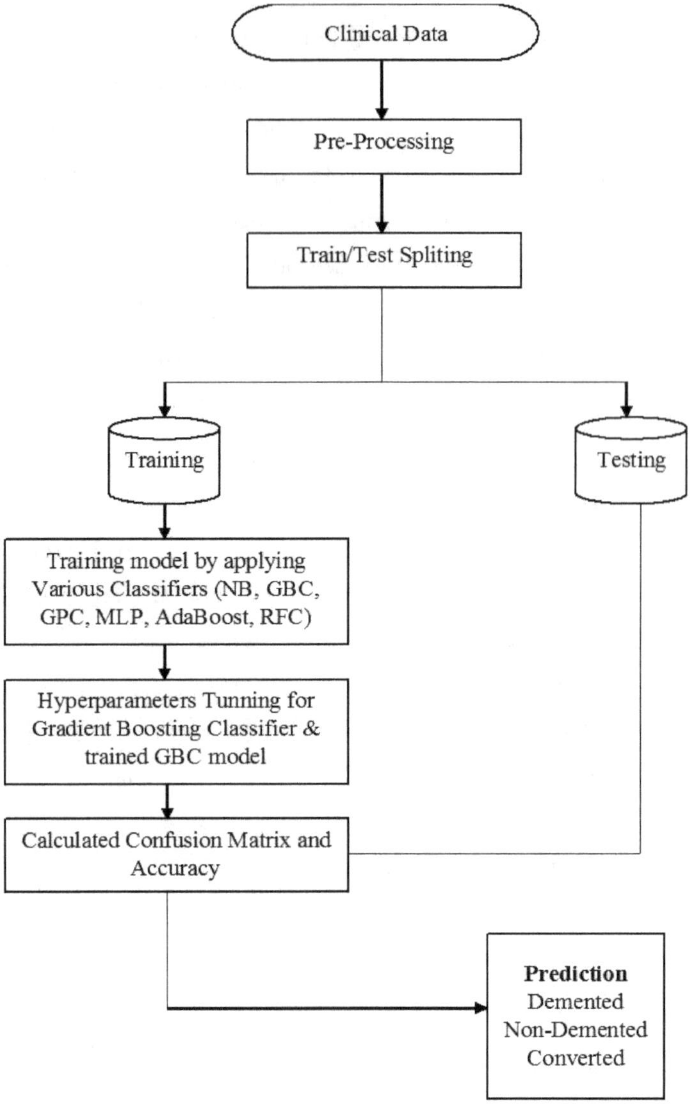

Fig. 6.1 Block Diagram for GBC-HPT

Naïve Bayes Classifiers (NB)

Naïve Bayes (NB) is an efficient technique [Mitchell.M 2017] for building classifiers. This technique is based on the principle that the feature value is independent of each other. The Bayes classifier model is a supervised learning model and has many practical applications due to its reliance on maximum likelihood-based parameter estimation. This model can work even does not assume Bayesian probability or does not use any Bayesian methods [Sharmila. R., 2018]. Despite these assumptions regarding parameters, Naïve Bayes classifiers were able to handle many complex real-world situations quite well. Bayes Classification can provide better performances even on small training samples. On the other hand, while the efficacy of Naïve Bayes classifiers was proved in [Zhang. H 2004], Bayes classification was outperformed in [Caruana.R 2006] by other classifiers such as boosted trees or random forests.

Gaussian Naïve Bayes:

It is customary to assume that the continuous data associated with each class obeys Gaussian distribution. Let x be a continuous attribute in the training data. This data may be first segmented by class value, and then the mean and variance of x may be computed for each class. Let $\mu_k$be the mean of the values in x associated with classC_k and let σ_k^2 be the variance of the values in x associated with classC_k. For the collected observation value v, the probability distribution $p(x = v|C_k)$ of v for given classC_k is computed using Eqn. (6.1)

$$P(x = v|C_k) = \frac{1}{\sqrt{2\pi\sigma_k}} e^{-\frac{1}{2}\left(\frac{v-\mu_k}{\sigma_k}\right)^2} \tag{6.1}$$

Multilayer Perceptrons (MLP)

A perceptron is a classification algorithm that divides the specified entry into two linear-functional categories known as a linear classifier [Iddamalgoda 2016]. Typically, the input is a vector x multiplied by weights w and added to it is a bias b, mathematically expressed as $w^T x + b$. Additionally, a perceptron sometimes passes $w^T x + b$ through a non-linear activation function y and deals with it in the form $y(w^T x + b)$.

Activation Function: In MLPs, neurons modeled after biological neurons are fired using non-linear activation functions. The two commonly used activation features are sigmoid and tanh. The sigmoid function is described in Eqn.(6.2), and tanh is described in Eqn. (6.3).

$$y(v_i) = tanh(v_i) \tag{6.2}$$

$$y(v_i) = \frac{1}{1+e^{-v_i}} \tag{6.3}$$

The hyperbolic tangent ranges in value from −1 to 1. The second function, referred to as the logistic function, has a shape similar to the hyperbolic tangent function but ranges in value from 0 to 1. Here $y(v_i)$ is the ith node's output in the input connections, and vi is the weighted sum. Other activation functions have also been proposed, such as Rectified Linear Unit, softmax function, and radial base features.

Multilayer Perceptrons (MLP) includes a layer of input and perhaps one or several hidden layers of nodes with activation functions that are non-linearly activated. MLPs are used to handle supervised learning problems. A given set of input-output pairs is used for training a model so that the correlations/dependencies/association between the inputs and outputs. During such modeling, the weights may need to be adjusted while training to minimize error. An iterative process typically adjusts the weights. There may be a need to adjust the weight to achieve the desired classification values through network training and dataset training.

Random Forest Classifier

The Random Forest Classifier (RFC) performs regression tasks as well as classification tasks using a supervised learning approach. It also performs dimensionality reduction and handles missing values, outliers, and other essential processes in data exploration, whenever needed. In the Ensemble learning method, a group of weak models aggregates to form a better-performing model efficient model [William Koehrsen 2019].

A Random Forest contains multiple trees, whereas the Classification and Regression Tree (CART) model involves a single tree. The trees in the forest participate in the classification by casting a vote for a class label to classify a new object. The class having the majority vote (by the trees in the forest) is selected as the class label for the object being classified. In regression, the forest takes the average value of the outputs provided by different trees as the needed result.

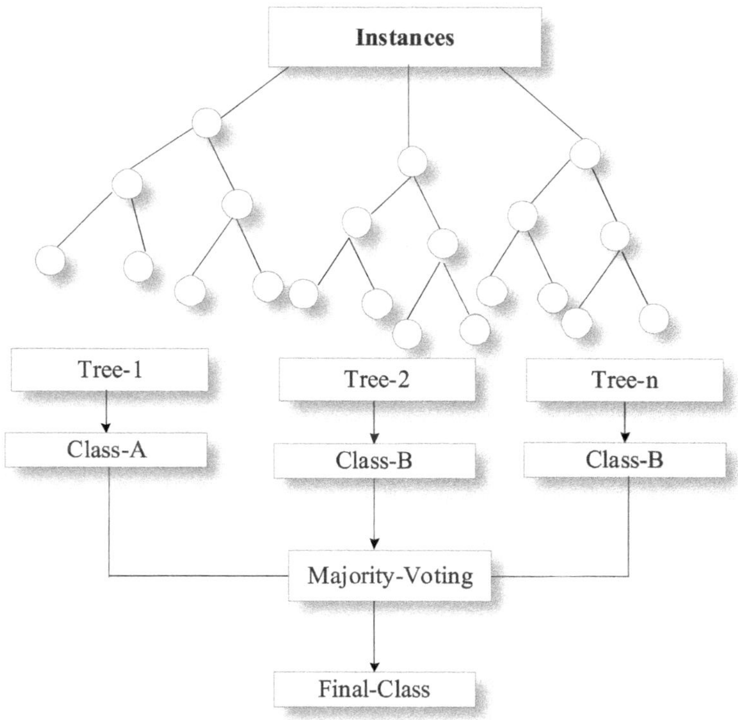

Fig. 6.2 Random Forest Classifier Model

Algorithm for Random Forest

In the first phase, the random forest algorithm chooses k from several m characteristics by random means. The root node with the best division approach can be found in phase two, with the randomly chosen k characteristics. The child nodes are calculated with the best-divided strategy in the third phase. The fourth phase is the repeat of the first three steps before the tree is formed on a root node with a target amount of leaf nodes. The four first phases are repeated in the last phase so that n trees are altered and thus, the random forest is formed.

6.1 Algorithmic Description of Random Forest

begin

1. From a total m features, k features are randomly selected (k <<m)
2. The root node is based on the k characteristics with the best strategy segmented
3. Divide the nodes into child nodes with the highest division.
4. Steps 1 through 3 will repeat until nodes are reached.
5. Steps 1 through 4 are repeated n times to create n trees.

End

6.3 GRADIENT BOOSTING CLASSIFIER WITH HYPERPARAMETER TUNING (GBC-HPT)

Two buzzwords, Bagging and Boosting, are frequently encountered while working with ensemble algorithms. The word bagging relates to creating learning algorithms on a random basis and determining the probabilities of bagging. On the other hand, the term boosting refers to a similar process, but sample selection is carried out more intelligently. This process assigns increasing weights to hard-to-classify observations [Grover Prince 2019].

The gradient boosting classifier does boost as opposed to bagging, and that is shown in fig. 6.3. This booster technique uses the logic in which subsequent forecasters learn from the errors of previous forecasters. The observations should be observed that they are not selected by bootstrap but are based on errors. Predictions can be selected from various models, such as decision trees, regression, and classification systems. The new predictions learn from prior prediction errors; it requires less time/phrases to approach the real predictions. However, the stopping criteria should be chosen carefully, or the process could lead to overfitting on training data.

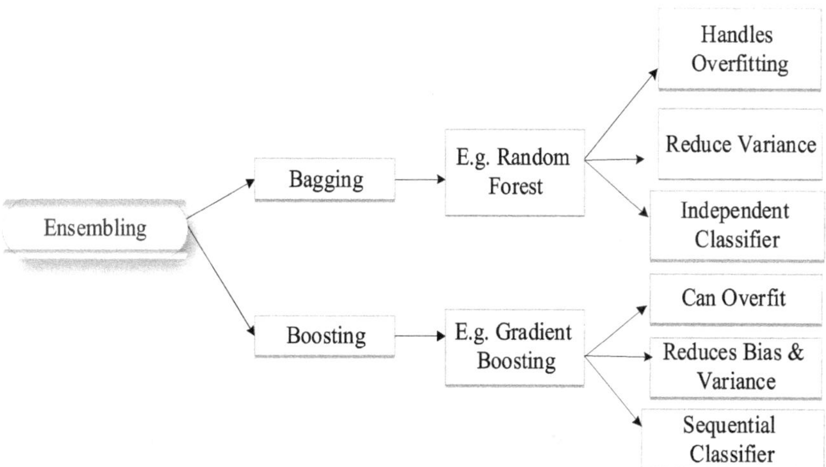

Fig. 6.3 Types of Ensemble Model

Gaussian Process Classifier (GPC)

Joint probability distribution and the Bayes rule form the basis for probabilistic classification. The Bayes theorem relates the joint probability and conditional probabilities of two stochastic events. Let x be the feature vector and y be the class label. Then, the Bayes theorem can be written as n shown in Eqn. (6.4)

$$p(y|x) = \frac{p(x,y)}{p(x)} = \frac{p(y).p(x|y)}{p(x)} \tag{6.4}$$

where $p(x|y)$ and $p(y|x)$are conditional probabilities, $p(x)$, and $p(y)$are prior probabilities of events x and y. Generative models find the posterior probability $p(y|x)$ for each class from the class's conditional probability and the prior probabilities. The generative model can be categorized into two types, namely *parametric* and *non-parametric*.

Gaussian Process Classifier is a non-parametric classification method that defines the posterior probabilities over a latent function $p(f)$ where the function $p(f)$ is assumed to be normal or Gaussian distribution. This assumption guarantees the smoothness of the underlying probability density function. It is subjected to a logistic likelihood function Ω like sigmoid function for classification. Let us consider a binary hypothesis deciding an entity to be either $C_1(y_i = 0)$ or $C_2(y_i = 1)$and x_i the feature vector of ith training sample with its class as C_j, where i varies from 1 to n; j is either 0 or 1; n is the number of training samples. This Gaussian process is characterized by the mean function $\mu(x)$and the covariance function $k(x, x')$.

$$k(x, x') = \sigma_j^2 \exp\left[-\frac{1}{2}\frac{(x-x')^2}{i^2}\right] \tag{6.5}$$

where σ_j^2 represents the maximum allowable covariance, and i represents the length parameter. If $k(x, x')$ is high, then it means that $f(x)$ *and* $f(x')$ are perfectly correlated. The Gaussian process classifier learns the hyperparameters from the training samples, computes the maximum likelihood, and makes posterior inference. Let x_{n+1}be a test feature vector with its corresponding latent variablef_{n+1}. The objective is to determine the class label y_{n+1}. The posterior probability for class$C_1$is given in Eqn. (6.6)

$$P(C_1|x) = P(y_i = 0|f_i) = \Omega(\mathrm{f_i(x)}) \tag{6.6}$$

First, the distribution of the test vector is calculated as

$$p(f_{n+1}|X, y, x_{n+1}) = \int p(f_{n+1}|X, y, x_{n+1}, f)p(f|X,)pdf \tag{6.7}$$

The computation of this distribution on the latent variable is later achieved by the f_{n+1} as

$$p(y_{n+1}|f_{n+1}) = \int \Omega(f_{n+1})p(f_{n+1}|X, y, x_{n+1}, f)df_{n+1} \tag{6.8}$$

The Laplace approximation and the projection propagation are two analytic approximations that use non-Gaussian posterior Gaussian joints. These can also be employed with the Gaussian process for classification.

Adaptive Boosting Classifier (AdaBoost)

A classifier AdaBoost fits a classifier into the initial dataset first. The same data set also contains extra copies of the classifier. In the second pass, AdaBoost adjusts the weights of wrongly categorized cases and concentrates more on complex cases (See Fig. 6.4).

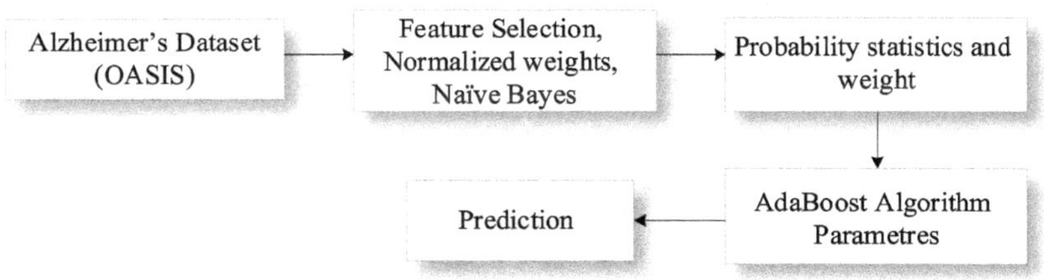

Fig. 6.4 Ada Booster Classifier Model

AdaBoost Classifier Hyperparameters:

1. ***base_estimator*: (data type: *object*; data value:max_depth:5)**

   The boosted ensemble is constructed using this estimator.

2. ***n_estimator*: (data type: *integer*; data value: 300)**

   Before boosting, the limits on the number of estimators are set. The learning process may stop soon if it is perfectly fit.

3. ***Learning_rate*:(data type: float; data value:0.001)**

   The learning rate shrinks the contribution of each classifier based on the given learning rate. There is a trade-off between learning rate and n estimators.

4. **algorithm: (data type: SAMME)**

   This parameter allows the choice between the discrete versus real boosting algorithm. When this parameter has a value 'SAMME.R', the real boosting algorithm is used, and the base estimator parameter is expected to support the calculation of class probabilities. The discrete boosting algorithm is used when ' SAMME ' is selected. Typically, the actual algorithm converges faster than the discrete algorithm and produces a reduced test mistake, and fewer iterations are required.

5. **random state: (data type: *integer*; data value: 60)**

   This parameter indicates information used for random number generation. When *int* is chosen for the random state, then it represents the seed that needs to be used by the random number generator. On the other hand, when Random State is chosen for a random state, it specifies the random number generator to be used.

6. **Feature_importances: (data type: SAMME; data values:7)**

   The impurity-based feature importance

6.2 Algorithmic Description for AD-GBC-HPT

Input: Clinical Data from MR Brain Images

Output: Classification of Alzheimer's Disease Stages

begin

Phase–I: Pre-Processing

Step 1: Read the Clinical Data

Step2: Data imputation for filing up missing values.

Step 3: Split Training and Testing Data

Phase –II: Classification

Step 4: Tuning the GBC hyperparameters

Step 5: Train the data using the GBC model

Step 6: Testing the Trained GBC model for Evaluation.

End

6.4 RESULTS AND DISCUSSION

The findings are given in this chapter obtained when the different classifiers are used on OASIS Dataset. The classification results are measured as Accuracy, Precision, Recall, and F1-Score. A discussion of results is also included in this section.

Table 6.1 Performance of Random Forest Classifier

Group	Precision	Recall	F1-Score
Converted	0.00	0.00	0.00
Demented	1.00	0.90	0.95
Non-demented	0.98	0.88	0.93
Avg	0.89	0.81	0.85

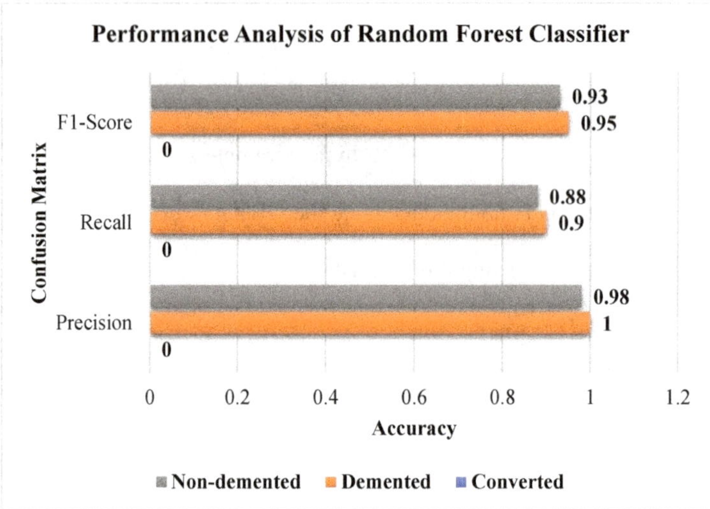

Fig. 6.5 Performance Analysis of Random Forest Classifier

Fig. 6.5 and Table 6.1 shows the performance of the Random Forest Classifier Model. This model's accuracy is 88%. It exhibits higher prediction performance on both Demented and the Non-Demented classes.

Table 6.2 Performance of Gradient Boosting Classifier with Hyperparameter Tuning

Group	Precision	Recall	F1-Score
Converted	0.50	1.00	0.67
Demented	1.00	0.92	0.96
Non-demented	0.98	0.93	0.95
Avg	0.93	0.94	0.93

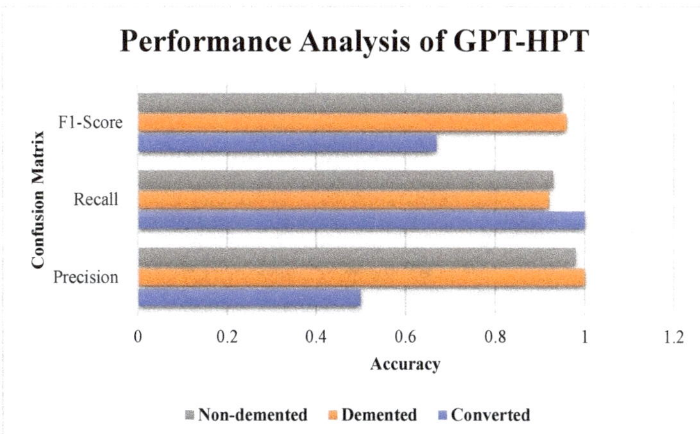

Fig. 6.6 Performance Analysis of Gradient Boosting Classifier with Hyperparameter Tuning

Table 6.2 and Fig. 6.6 show the Gradient Boosting Classifier's performance with the hyperparameters tuning (GBC-HPT) model. Its classification accuracy is 96%, which is 8% more than the Random Forest classifier. Further, the model was able to identify all the three classes, making it one of the best classifiers in the current analysis.

Table 6.3 Performance of Gaussian Processing Classifier

Group	Precision	Recall	F1-Score
Converted	0.00	0.00	0.00
Demented	0.81	0.93	0.87
Non-demented	0.97	0.79	0.87
Avg	0.84	0.80	0.81

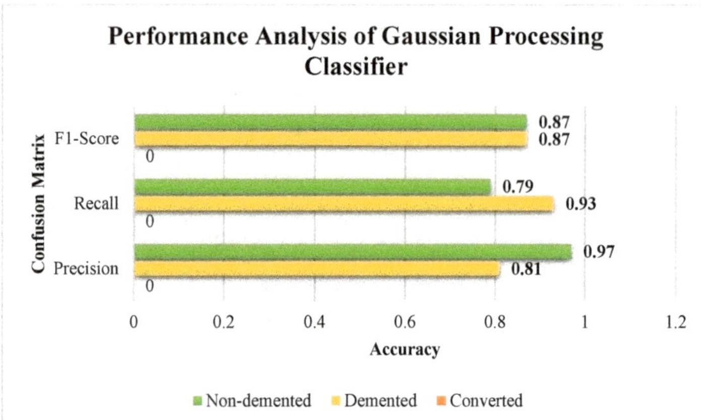

Fig. 6.7 Performance Analysis of Gaussian Processing Classifier

Fig. 6.7 and Table 6.3 shows the Gaussian Processing Classifier (GPC) model. Performance values for this model show that classification accuracy is 77.33%. This model exhibits good precision values; however, the recall levels were found to be lower compared to other models.

Table 6.4 Performance Analysis of Naïve Bayes Classifier

Group	Precision	Recall	F1-Score
Converted	0.00	0.00	0.00
Demented	0.36	0.36	0.36
Non-demented	0.60	0.55	0.57
Avg	0.45	0.42	0.43

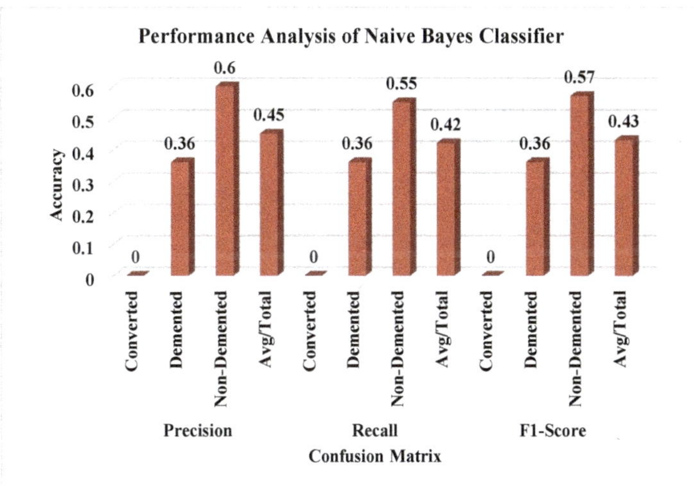

Fig. 6.8 Performance Analysis of Naïve Bayes Classifier

Table 6.4 and Fig. 6.8 show the performance measures of the Naïve Bayes Classifier (NBC) model. The accuracy of the model is 91.07%. Although the overall accuracy is high, specific class prediction levels are low.

Table 6.5 Performance Analysis of AdaBoost Classifier

Group	Precision	Recall	F1-Score
Converted	0.08	0.03	0.04
Demented	0.45	0.39	0.41
Non-demented	0.33	0.61	0.43
Avg	0.34	0.46	0.38

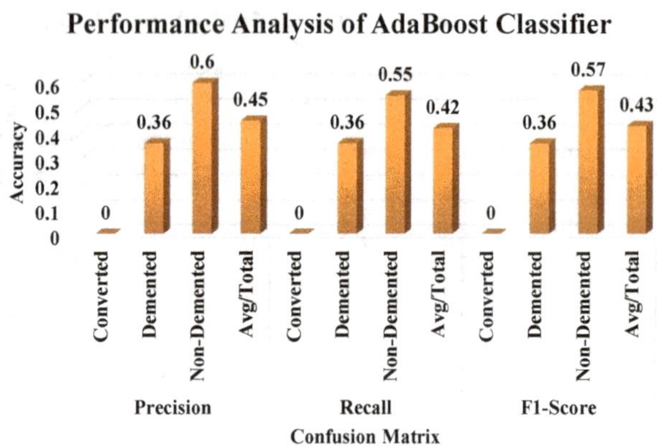

Fig. 6.9 Performance Analysis of AdaBoost Classifier

Fig. 6.9 and Table 6.5 shows the results of the AdaBoost Classifier model, with an accuracy of 66.96%. Although the model exhibits low performance compared to the other models, the model could predict all three classes compared to the other models, which were not effective on the classification of the Converted class.

Table 6.6 Performance Analysis of Multi-Layer Perception Classifier

Group	Precision	Recall	F1-Score
Converted	0.11	0.10	0.11
Demented	0.32	0.30	0.31
Non-demented	0.54	0.58	0.56
Avg	0.41	0.43	0.42

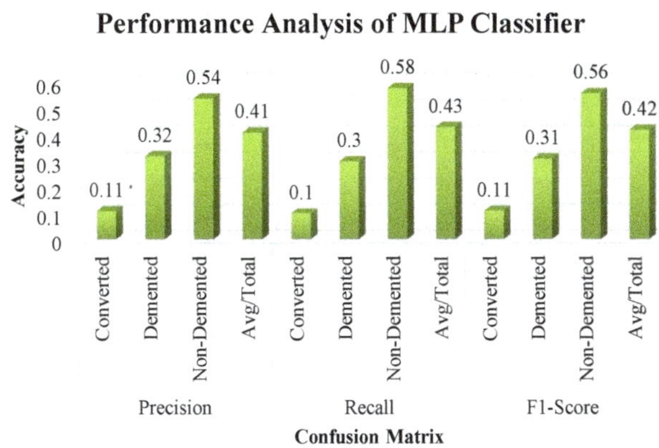

Fig 6.10 Performance Analysis of MLP Classifier

Table 6.6 and Fig. 6.10 shows the experimental results recorded for Multi-Layer Perception (MLP) Classifier model. The classification accuracy of this model is 40%. Even with low prediction performances, the model could effectively distinguish between the three classes, and thus confirms its suitability for classification.

Table 6.7 Precision Values of Classifiers

Group	RFC	GBC-HPT	GPC	NB	AdaBoost	MLP
Converted	0.00	**0.50**	0.00	0.00	0.08	0.11
Demented	1.00	**1.00**	0.81	0.36	0.45	0.32
Non-demented	0.98	**0.98**	0.97	0.60	0.33	0.54
Avg	0.89	**0.93**	0.84	0.45	0.34	0.41

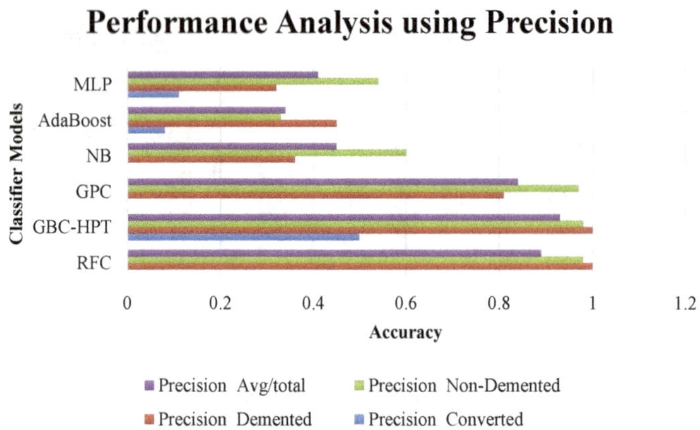

Fig. 6.11 Performance Analysis using Precision

Fig. 6.11 and Table 6.7 show the model-wise comparison of the six chosen models' classification potential as Precision values. It could be observed that MGBC exhibits the best performance in terms of class prediction and overall prediction, making it the most suitable model for this domain.

Table 6.8 Recall Values of Classifiers

Group	RFC	GBC-HPT	GPC	NB	AdaBoost	MLP
Converted	0.00	1.00	0.00	0.00	0.03	0.10
Demented	0.90	0.92	0.93	0.36	0.39	0.30
Non-demented	0.88	0.93	0.79	0.55	0.61	0.58
Avg	0.81	0.94	0.80	0.42	0.46	0.43

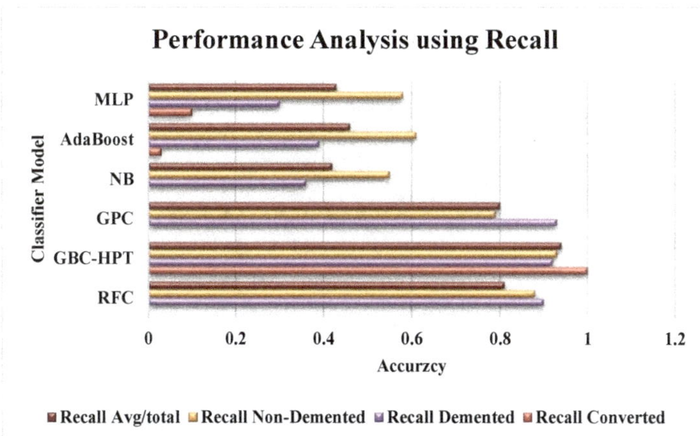

Fig. 6.12 Performance Analysis using Recall

Table 6.8 shows the classification efficiency of the mentioned six models in terms of Recall values. Fig.6.12 visualizes the accuracy of classification for those models, for the Recall values. Among those models, the GBC-HPT outperforms all the other models, qualifying itself as the most effective model.

Table 6.9 F1-Score Values of Classifiers

Group	RFC	GBC-HPT	GPC	NB	AdaBoost	MLP
Converted	0.00	0.67	0.00	0.00	0.04	0.11
Demented	0.95	0.96	0.87	0.36	0.41	0.31
Non-demented	0.93	0.95	0.87	0.57	0.43	0.56
Avg/total	0.85	0.93	0.81	0.43	0.38	0.42

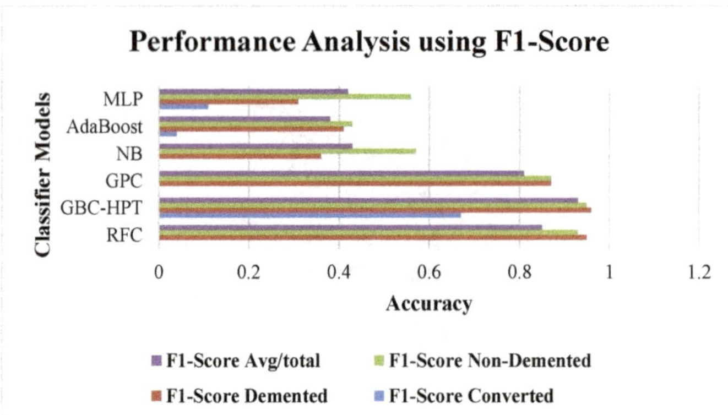

Fig. 6.13 Performance Analysis using F1-Score

The results obtained for the chosen six classification models on the F1-Score are furnished in Table 6.10. The comparative analysis of the results is shown in Fig.6.14. Among those methods, GBC-HPT scores better its competitive models.

Table 6.10 Accuracy of Classifiers

Group	RFC	GBC-HPT	GPC	NB	AdaBoost	MLP
Accuracy (%)	88	96	77.33	91.07	66.96	40

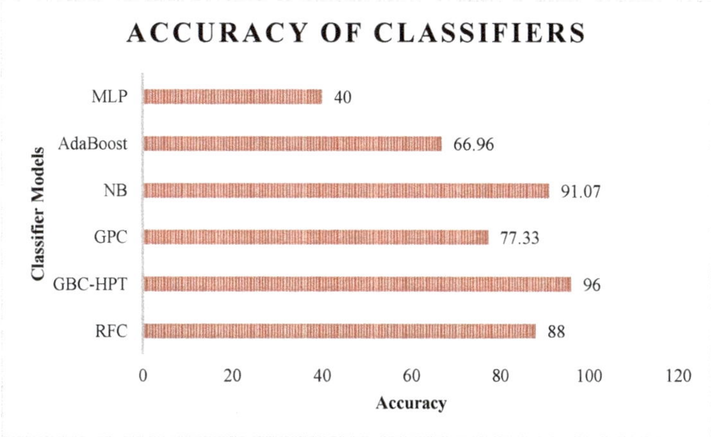

Fig. 6.14 Accuracy of Classifiers

Fig. 6.14 and Table 6.10 shows a comparison of the accuracy obtained by the various classifiers. AD-GBC-HPT exhibits the highest accuracy levels than all the other models, making it the best choice for operating on medical data.

The six quality indicators for the overall performance assessment of those chosen classifiers are Scant, Poor, Low, Moderate, High, and Excellent. Each classifier exhibits a certain level of performance, as listed below.

S: Scant performance if value achieved is 0–9%;

P: Poor performance if value achieved is 10–29%;

L: Low performance if value achieved is 30–49%;

M: Moderate performance if value achieved is 50–69%;

H: High performance if value achieved is 70–89%;

E: Excellent performance if value achieved is 90–100%

Table 6.11 Performance Summary of the Classifiers

Classifier \ Metric	Precision			Recall			F1-Score		
	C	**D**	**ND**	**C**	**D**	**ND**	**C**	**D**	**ND**
RFC	S	E	H	S	E	E	S	E	E
GBC	E	E	E	M	E	E	M	E	E
GPC	S	E	H	S	H	E	S	H	H
NB	S	L	M	S	L	M	S	L	M
AdaBoost	S	L	M	S	L	L	S	L	L
MLP	P	L	M	P	L	M	S	L	M
C: Converted; D: Demented; ND: Non-Demented **Excellent (E): 90-100; High (H): 70-89; Moderate (M): 50-69;** **Low (L): 30-49; Poor (P) 10-29; Scant (S): 0-9**									

Table 6.11 summarizes the information for six different classifiers using three different metrics (Precision, Recall, and F1-Score) for the three classes (Converted, Demented, and Non-Demented). A single classifier performing at an excellent level in one metric for a class may not perform well in the same metric for a different class. To visualize the above data for aside-by-side comparison of the classifiers, it assigns a quality index for the performance. It uses a 6-point scale having values 1 through 6 for the performance levels - Scant through Excellent. As an illustration, Fig. 6.15 shows the Precision values as the performance measure of different classifiers with three classes.

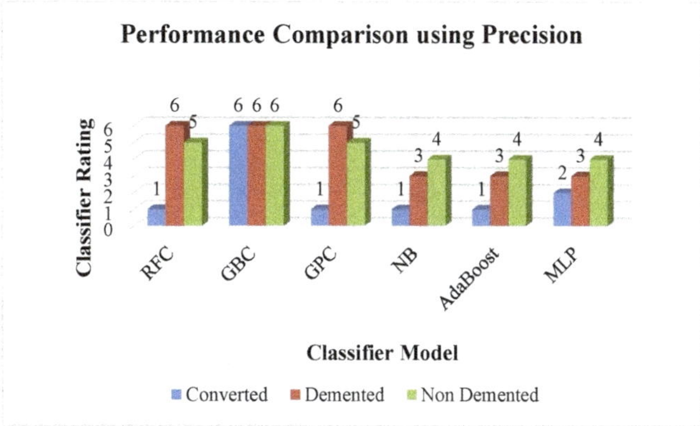

Fig. 6.15 Performance Comparison using Precision

Similarly, Fig. 6.16 compares the performance of the different classifiers when the metric used is Recall.

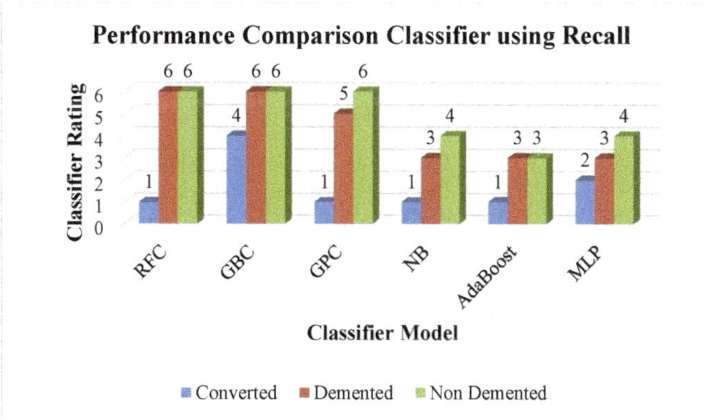

Fig. 6.16 Performance Comparison of Classifiers using Recall

Finally, Fig. 6.17 compares the performance of the different classifiers when using the F1-Score metric.

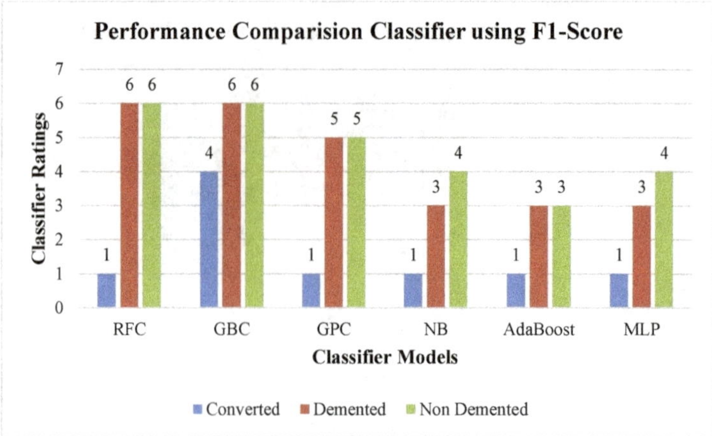

Fig. 6.17 Performance Comparison of Classifiers in F1-Score

GBC and GPC are Excellent for Demented classification, whereas GBC alone is Excellent on non-demented and on Converted. When the metrics of Recall and F1-Score are used, RFC and GBC exhibit excellent performance for demented and Non-Demented classes. On the other hand, on the Converted classification, except GBC, these classifiers uniformly exhibit scant or poor performance. It is evident that GBC consistently outperforms its counterparts in the classification of Converted, Demented, and Non-Demented, while NB, AdaBoost, and MLP are observed to perform far below average. Based on the results presented in Table 6.11, it can also be inferred that GBC outperforms the rest of the classifiers. GBC's excellent performance is attributed to the process of boosting in GBC that ideally helps to minimize overfitting, bias, and variance.

6.5 DECISION TREE CLASSIFIER ALGORITHM WITH HYPERPARAMETER TUNING (AD-DTC-HPT)

The proposed method handles the pre-processed data and applies the feature extraction process. Those features are used to optimize the decision tree for AD classification. DTC-HPT approach is a tree-based classification model and is processed compared to the decision tree classifier to classify AD stages. It is also evident that the accuracy of prediction/classification of clinical data is duly affected by various pre-processing elements, such as data imputation and feature selection. To provide feasible solutions for this research work proposes a new mechanism for the imperative classification of AD from clinical Alzheimer's datasets using a Decision Tree Classifier with hyperparameter tuning (AD-DTC-HPT).

6.5.1 METHODOLOGY OF AD-DTC-HPT

Decision tree classification is a traditional data classification technique that has several applications. Decision trees are constructed in numerous ways as branch-like fragments. The decision tree starts with a root node; leaf nodes denote the class labels, while the intermediate nodes are referred to as non-leaf / child nodes. The data attribute with the highest priority in decision making is chosen as the root node. The splitting process of a decision tree is decided upon the respective node [Han.J.2011]. In this method, four vital attributes contribute to a higher probability of detecting AD. They are Gender (G), Age (A), Hand (H), Mini-Mental State Examination (MMSE), and Clinical Dementia Ratio (CDR). These attributes represent the critical factors that have a bearing on developing AD.

In machine learning, the decision tree classifier learns during the training phase, and the effectiveness of the classifier is assessed during the testing phase. The decision tree depth and the distribution of training and test information are variables that influence the performance and effectiveness of the classifier. The hyperparameters for the Decision tree classifier are listed below.

A. ***max:*** **(data type: *integer*; data value: 7)**

   The tree node's maximum depth is extended to cover all sheets pure or to allow all sheets to contain less than min samples split samples.

B. **Criterion: (data type: *string;* data value: 'Gini', 'Entropy')**

   The estimation function of a divided quality. The criteria supported are "gini" for the Gini impurity and "entropy."

C. **splitter: (data type: *string;* data value: 'random')**

   The strategy used for dividing every node. Strategies supported are "best" to choose the best division and the best random division to select.

D. **min samples split: (data type: *string;* data value: 5)**

The minimum amount for dividing an inner node: If int, consider the minimum amount of min samples split. For minimum samples split, the minimum sample number of each split, if floating, is a fraction and the ceiling (min samples split * n samples).

E. **max Leaf nodes: (data type: *integer;* data value: 9)**

Develop a tree in the best fashion with max leaf nodes. If None, the number of nodes will be unlimited.

F. **max features: (data type: *integer;* data value: 4)**

- The number of functions to consider when searching for the best division:
- If int, consider the max features at each division.
- If float is a fraction of max features and int (max features*n features) is taken into account in every division. If "auto", then max_features=sqrt(n_features).
- MAX features = sqrt(n features) if "sqrt"
- If "log2," max features = log2(n features) will be used.
- If none, then max function = n functionality.

G. **min_impurity_decrease: (data type: *float;* data value: 0.5)**

A node splits if this split induces a decrease of the impurity greater than or equal to this value.

H. **min_impurity_split: (data type: *float;* data value: 0.20)**

It is the threshold for early stopping during tree growth. A node will split if its impurity is above the threshold, and otherwise, it is a leaf.

The Block diagram of the AD-DTC-HPT Classifier Model is shown in Fig. 6.18

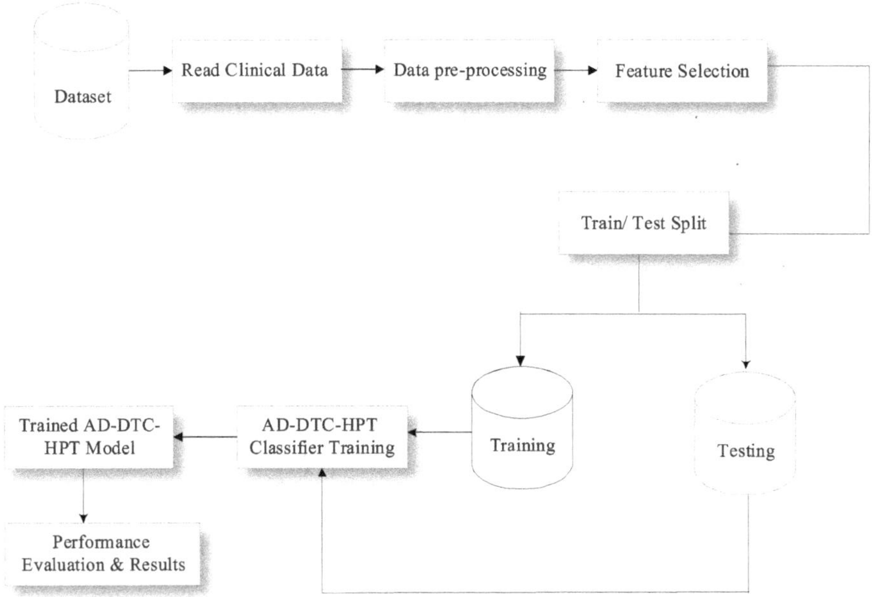

Fig. 6.18 Block Diagram of AD-DTC-HPT Classifier Model

6.3 Algorithmic Descriptions for AD-DTC-HPT

Input: Clinical Data from MRI Brain images

Output: Classification of Alzheimer's Disease Stages

Proposed AD-DTC-HPT method

begin

Phase I: Pre-Processing

Step 1: Read the clinical data

Step 2: Pre-Process using Data Imputation for filling in the missing values

Step 3: Perform One-hot Encoding

Phase II: Classification

Step 4: Split data for Training and Testing

Step 5: On training, apply DTC-HPT classifier Algorithm

Step 6: Classifier algorithm computes the information of D as

$$info(D) = -\sum_{i=1}^{m} p_i log_2(p_i) \quad (6.3.1)$$

where p_i is the probability of prediction groups, i.

Step 7: The information and gain of the imputed dataset, DI is computed as

$$info_x(DI) = \sum_{i=1}^{x} \frac{|D_j|}{|D|} \times I(DI_j) \quad (6.3.2)$$

where information gain i is an attribute of DI

$$Gain(X) = info(D) - info \quad (DI) \quad (6.3.3)$$

(The attribute that gives us the highest gain is used as the splitting attribute.)

Step 8: Evaluate the Performance of the proposed Classifier Algorithm using the Test dataset.

end

Estimated Total Intracranial Volume (eTIV) and Normalized Whole-brain Volume (nWBV)

To produce cortical and sub-cortical measures, [Alexander Bernstein 2018] pipeline is used for Free Surfer. In this research, Free Surfer produced an estimated total Intracranial volume (eTIV) for Internal Cerebral Vein (ICV). The eTIV measure from Free Surfer complies with the fractionation of Internal Cerebral Vein (ICV) references obtained from the weighted proton density images. The pipeline produced 68 cortical volumes and 46 sub-cortical volumes

(34 from each hemisphere). Further assessment excluded white matter hypogene, optical chiasm, left and right choroidal plexus, and left and right choroid plexus. Cortical and subcortical volumetric measurements were averaged on the right and the left. For the final analysis, the research utilized 34 regional cortical volumes and 17 sub-cortical volumes. The visually inspected steps ensure that the feature extractions (skull stripping faults and gray/white matter boundary).

6.6 RESULTS AND DISCUSSION

Different classifiers were trained using the dataset, and the performance metrics, namely Precision, Accuracy, Recall, F1-Score, were determined for each classifier. The results presented here will provide a comparison of the performance of the Decision Tree classifiers concerning each metric.

Table 6.12 Performance of DTC (with Missing Values)

Group	**Precision**	**Recall**	**F1-Score**	**Support**
Mild AD	0.13	0.17	0.15	12
Moderate AD	0.00	0.00	0.00	2
Non-demented	0.54	0.63	0.58	59
Very Mild AD	0.29	0.21	0.24	39
Classification Report				
Macro Avg	0.24	0.25	0.24	112
Weighted Avg	0.40	0.42	0.40	112
Accuracy: 0.41964285714285715 (41.96%)				

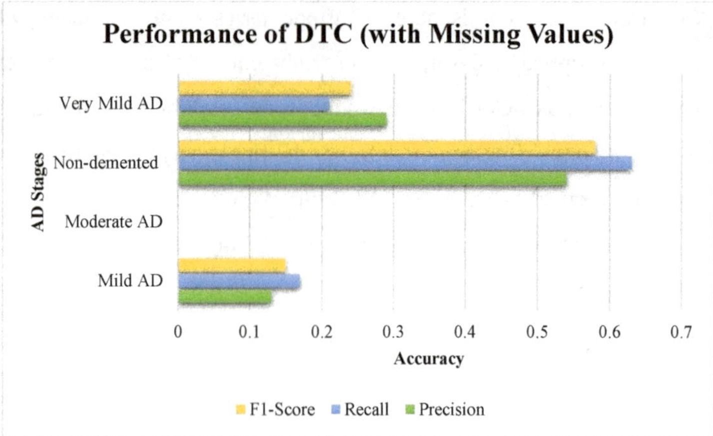

Fig. 6.19 Performance Analysis of DTC with Missing Values

Table 6.12 and Fig. 6.19 show the missing data without data imputation using the DTC classifier model. The DTC classifier model performance values for the chosen metrics. The accuracy of the model is 41.96%. The table shows the deficient performance of the model before the imputation process.

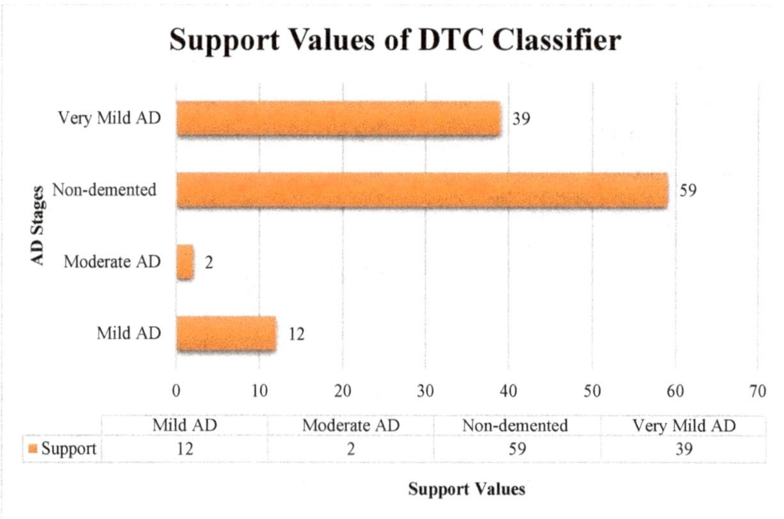

Fig. 6.20 Support Values of DTC

Table 6.13 Performance of DTC (with Data Imputation)

Group	Precision	Recall	F1-Score	Support
Mild AD	0.25	0.22	0.24	9
Moderate AD	0.00	0.00	0.00	1
Non-demented	0.71	0.59	0.65	76
Very Mild AD	0.23	0.35	0.27	26
Classification Report				
Macro Avg	0.30	0.29	0.29	112
Weighted Avg	0.56	0.50	0.52	112
Accuracy: 0.5 (50%)				

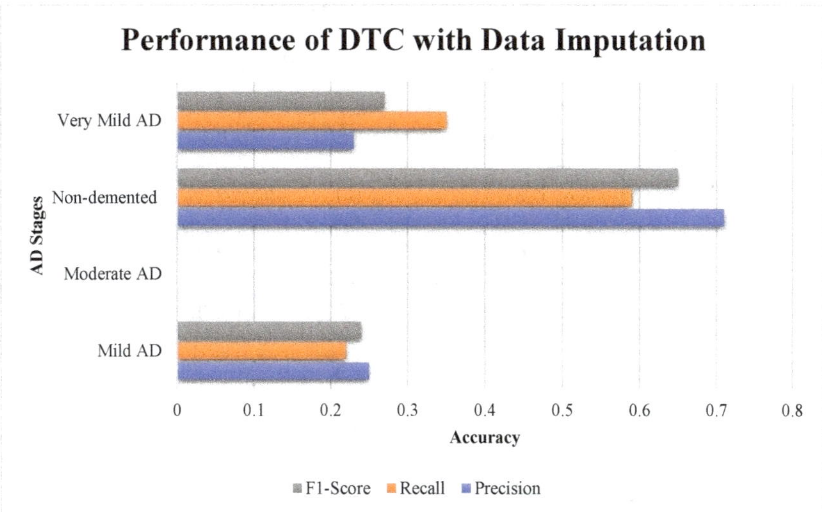

Fig. 6.21 Performance of DTC with Data Imputation

Table 6.13 and Fig. 6.21 shows the missing data with data imputation using DTC. The DTC classifier model performance values for the chosen metrics. The model accuracy is 50%. Imputation is performed using Mode, and a slight increase in performance in terms of all the metrics could be observed.

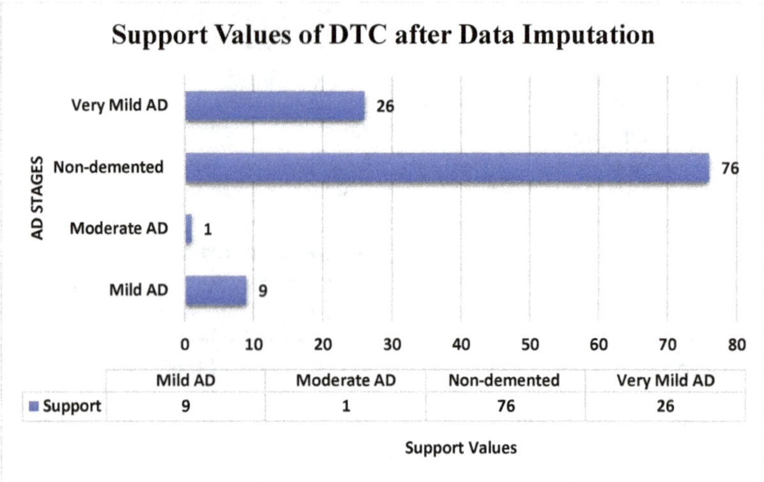

Fig. 6.22 Support Values of DTC after Data Imputation

Table 6.14 Performance Analysis of DTC - HPT

Group	Precision	Recall	F1-Score	Support
Mild AD	0.89	1.00	0.94	8
Moderate AD	0.00	0.00	0.00	1
Non-demented	1.00	1.00	1.00	63
Very Mild AD	1.00	1.00	1.00	40
Classification Report				
Macro Avg	0.72	0.75	0.74	112
Weighted Avg	0.98	0.99	0.99	112
Accuracy: 0.9910714285714286 (99.10%)				

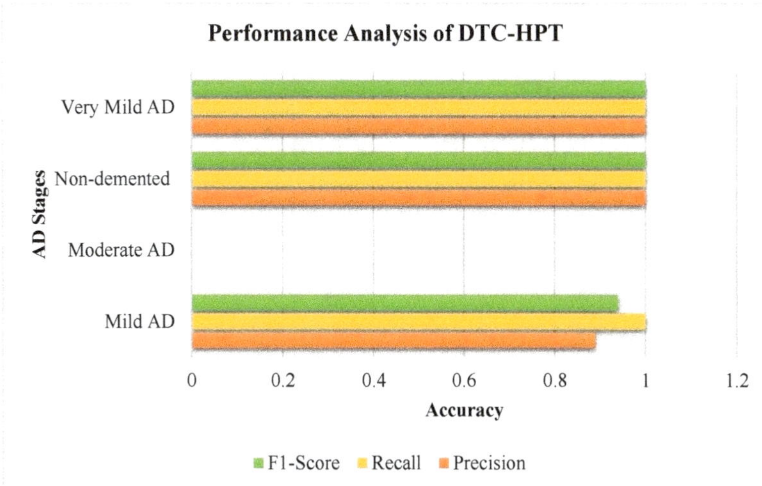

Fig. 6.23 Performance Analysis of DTC-HPT

Fig. 6.23 and Table 6.14 shows the performance MDTC classifier model performance values for the chosen metrics. The model accuracy is 99.10%. A boost of 50% could be observed after tuning of the hyperparameters. This shows the efficiency of the tuning process.

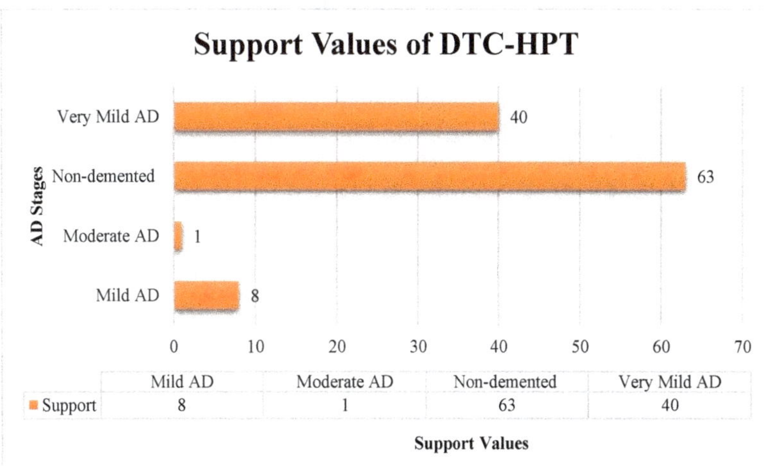

Fig. 6.24 Support Values of DTC-HPT

Table 6.15 Feature Importance of Clinical Data Columns (DTC)

Clinical Data Columns	Feature Importance
Visit	2.69%
Gender	0.00%
Hand	16.05%
Age	6.53%
SES	6.33%
MMSE	5.92%
eTIV	19.64%
nWBV	15.55%
ASF	0.00%
EDUC	1.04%
MR Delay	5.55%
CDR	20.69%

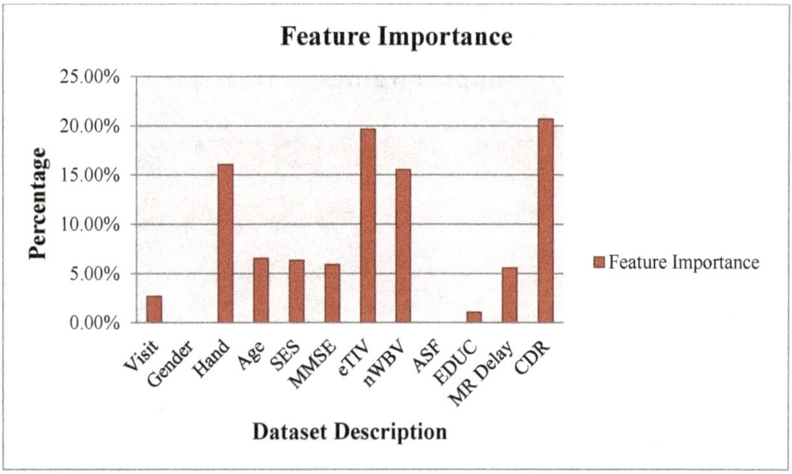

Fig. 6.25 Feature Importance in DTC Model

Table 6.15 and Fig. 6.25 show the feature importance of Decision Tree Classifier (DTC) before the modification proposed in DTC-HPT, and Table 6.16 and Fig. 6.26 shows the feature importance of the DTC-HPT model.

Table 6.16 Feature Importance of Clinical Data Columns (DTC-HPT)

Clinical Data Columns	Feature Importance
Visit	0.00%
Gender	0.00%
Hand	0.00%
Age	0.00%
SES	0.00%
MMSE	6.33%
eTIV	0.00%
nWBV	0.00%
ASF	0.00%
EDUC	1.15%
MR Delay	1.69%
CDR	97.16%

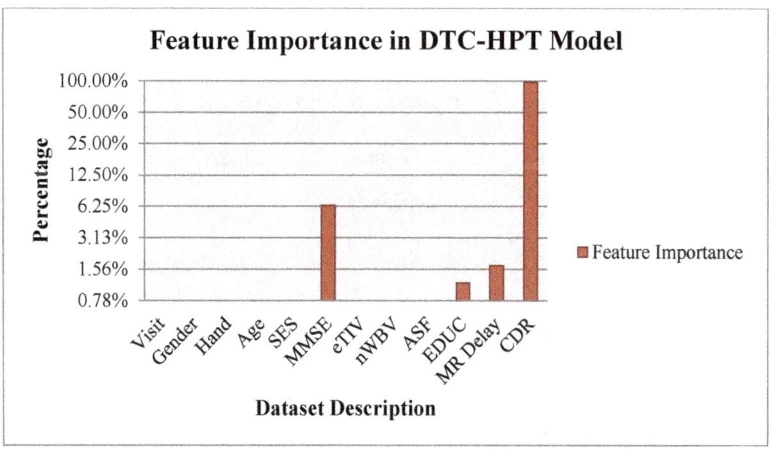

Fig. 6.26 Feature Importance in DTC-HPT Model

Table 6.17 Comparison of Accuracy after Data imputation

Method	Accuracy
DTC	50%
DTC-HPT	99.10%

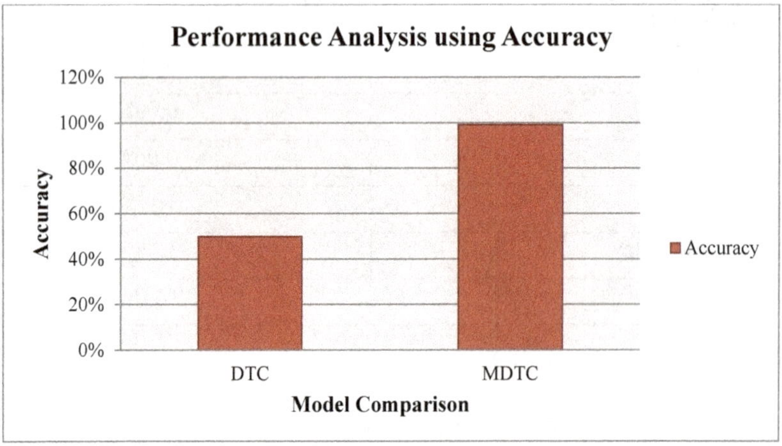

Fig. 6.27 Performance Analysis using Accuracy

Fig. 6.27 and Table 6.17 show the comparison of Accuracy of the two methods Decision Tree Classifier (DTC) and Decision Tree Classifier tuning hyperparameter (DTC-HPT). It could be observed that the modified decision tree exhibits a ~50% increase in performance. The results show that the proposed model has high prediction potential.

Table 6.18 Comparison of Accuracy

Method	Accuracy
DTC with Missing Data	41.96%
DTC after Data Imputation	50%
DTC-HPT	99.10%

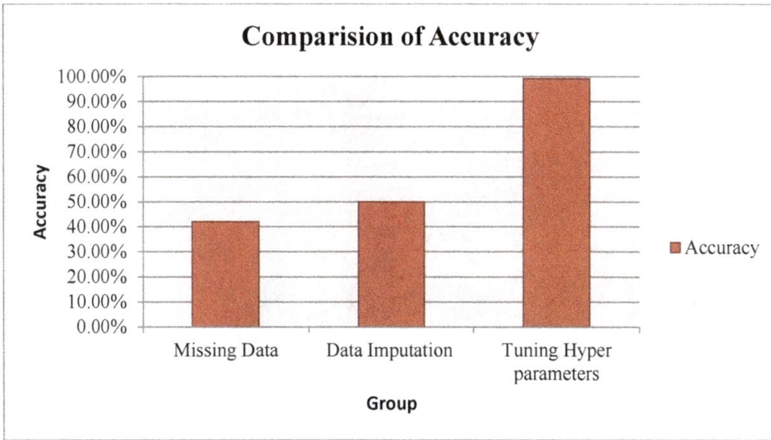

Fig. 6.28 Comparison Analysis using Accuracy

An increase in performance efficiency is evidenced in Table 6.18 by tuning the parameters. After every modification, an improvement in performance is observed.

Table 6.19 Comparison of Support

Group	DTC with Missing Value	DTC after Data Imputation	DTC-HPT
Mild AD	12	9	8
Moderate AD	2	1	1
Non-Demented	59	76	63
Very Mild AD	39	26	40

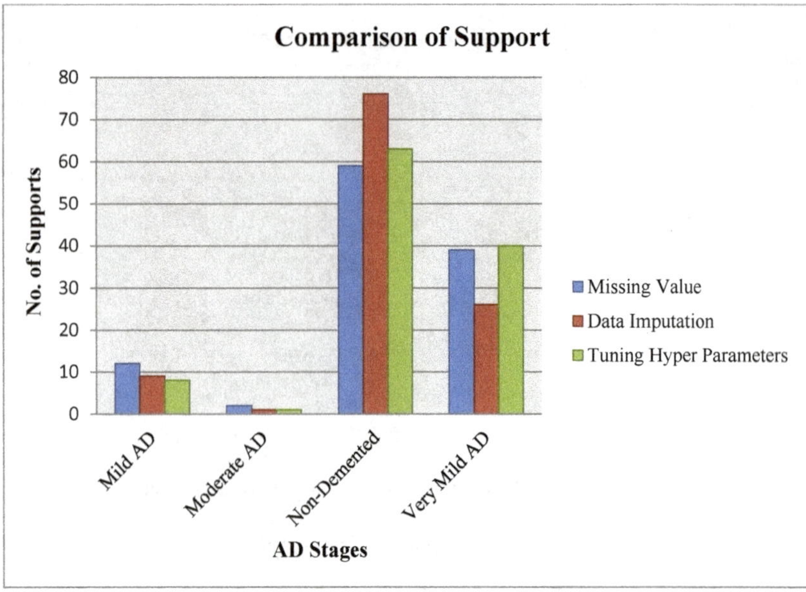

Fig. 6.29 Comparison of Support

A comparison analysis in Tables 6.19 and fig. 6.28 shows improved performance levels between DTC and DTC-HPT. The performance improvement is explicit, showing the efficiency of the model.

Table 6.20 Comparison of Precision

Group	DTC with Missing Value	DTC after Data Imputation	DTC-HPT
Mild AD	0.13	0.25	0.89
Moderate AD	0.00	0.00	0.00
Non-Demented	0.54	0.71	1.00
Very Mild AD	0.29	0.23	1.00

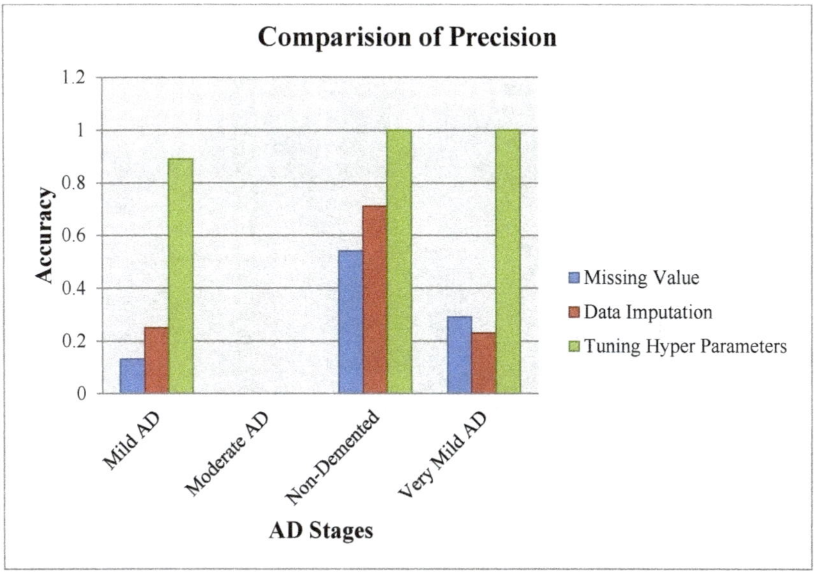

Fig. 6.30 Comparison of Precision

A comparison analysis of Precision in Tables 6.20 and fig. 6.29 shows improved performance levels between DTC and DTC-HPT. The performance improvement is explicit, showing the efficiency of the model.

Table 6.21: Comparison Analysis of Recall

Group	DTC with Missing Value	DTC after Data Imputation	DTC-HPT
Mild AD	0.17	0.22	1.00
Moderate AD	0.00	0.00	0.00
Non-Demented	0.63	0.59	1.00
Very Mild AD	0.21	0.35	1.00

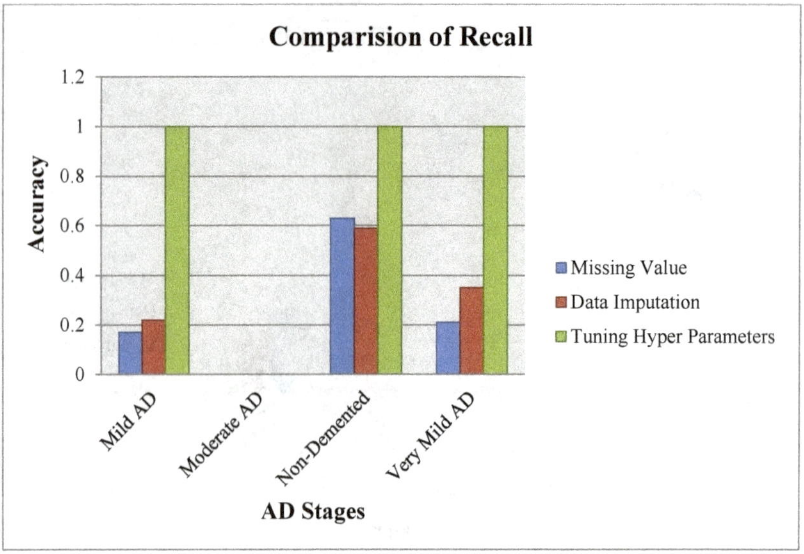

Fig. 6.31 Comparison of Recall

Performance comparison analysis using Recall in Tables 6.21 and Fig. 6.30 shows improved performance levels between DTC and DTC-HPT. The performance improvement is explicit, showing the efficiency of the model.

Table 6.22 Comparison of F1-Score

Group	DTC with Missing Value	DTC after Data Imputation	DTC-HPT
Mild AD	0.15	0.24	0.94
Moderate AD	0.00	0.00	0.00
Non-Demented	0.58	0.65	1.00
Very Mild AD	0.24	0.27	1.00

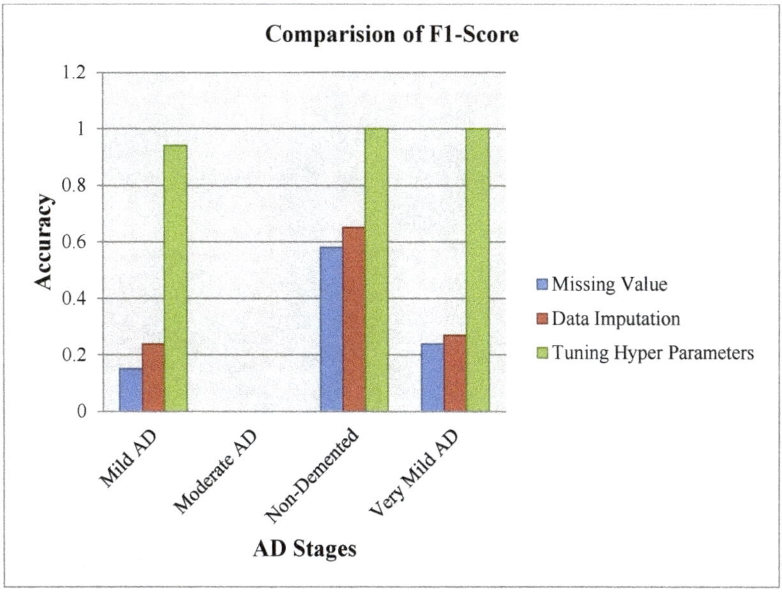

Fig. 6.32 Comparison of F1-Score

Performance comparison analysis using F1-Score in Tables 6.22 and fig. 6.30 shows the improvement in performance levels between DTC and DTC-HPT. The performance improvement is explicit, showing the efficiency of the model.

Table 6.23: Comparison of Support Values

Classifier	Mild AD	Moderate AD	Non-Demented	Very Mild AD
DTC	9	1	64	33
AD-DTC-HPT	13	1	67	37

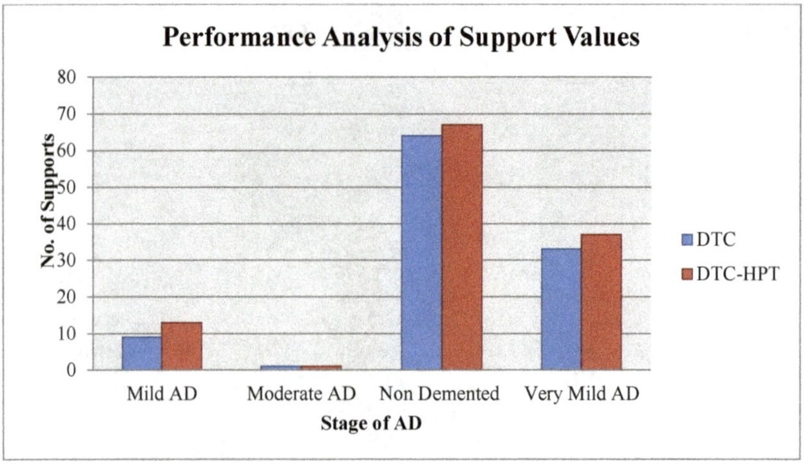

Fig. 6.33 Performance Analysis of Support Values

Performance comparison analysis using Support in Tables 6.23 and fig. 6.32 shows improved performance levels between DTC and AD-DTC-HPT. The performance improvement is explicit, showing the efficiency of the model.

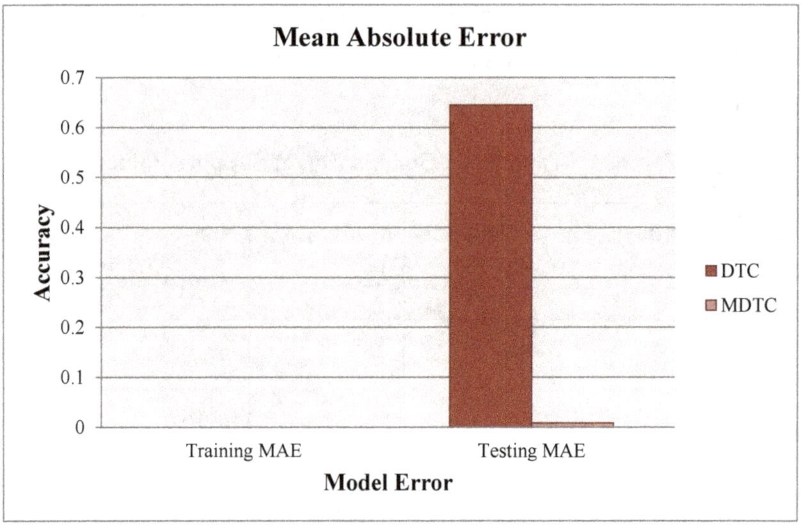

Fig. 6.34 Mean Absolute Error (MAE) on Training and Testing Data

A comparative analysis for Mean Absolute Error in fig. 6.34 shows improved performance levels between DTC and AD-DTC-HPT. The performance improvement is explicit, showing the efficiency of the model.

6.7 CONCLUSION

Rather than discovering a cure, more attention is paid to the decrease of risks, early intervention, and prompt dementia diagnosis in older adults. The literature study demonstrated early detection of AD using different machine learning algorithms and micro-simulation methods. However, identifying appropriate characteristics, which could assist in identifying dementia at an early stage, is still highly necessary.

Decision Tree Classification with the hyperparameter Tuning (AD-DTC-HPT) technique is a new methodology to detect AD at the early stages. It develops a Decision tree dependent on a preparation set that addresses an example of clinical information. It uses Entropy and Information Gain to figure out which credit to branch at each tree's dimension. Utilizing Information Gain empowers to build an ideal or close ideal tree with lesser nodes and branches than if resorts to an irregular determination of traits. Finally, once a Decision tree is built, the framework can anticipate new patients' circumstances concerning AD. The Decision tree is crossed from the root hub downwards dependent on the new patients' ascribed values till a leaf node. The leaf node speaks to the forecast of AD involvement. It is confident that the decision tree needs to be rebuilt or refreshed periodically to incorporate information based on additional patients with established AD. This proposed word of AD-DTC-HPT technique would aid in refining the decision tree to increase the Precision further and helps in predicting true positive AD diagnosis with a higher degree of confidence in the future, thus increasing its clinical utility as an adjunct to the visual interpretation of MR brain images in the overall management of AD patients. Moreover, this technique can also be applied equally and effectively in other molecular imaging modalities such as PET and Functional MR (fMRI) imaging.

CHAPTER 7

ENSEMBLE BASED CLASSIFICATION OF ALZHEIMER'S DISEASE

7.1 INTRODUCTION

Early diagnosis of Alzheimer's Disease (AD) plays a vital role in deciding the suitable course of action. This research work reports on an ensemble classifier model for the diagnosis of AD. A new composite and comprehensive classification schemes for MRI termed as Alzheimer's disease analysis using Ensemble Classifier (AD-EC) of Machine Learning Model is developed. This ensemble stacking classifier is designed to build on the combination of five distinct methods Extra Tree Classifier (ETC), k-Nearest Neighbor (kNN), Support Vector Machine (SVM), Extreme Gradient Boosting (XGB), and Gradient Boosting Machine (GBM). In single or combined, these processes' performance is evaluated on a T1-weighted MRI image set of the Open Access Image Studies Series (OASIS) dataset. Precision, Recall, F1-Score, and Accuracy were recorded in the results. The performance of the stacked ensemble model is confirmed to outperform its counterparts progressively. The improved accuracy of ensemble classifiers experimented in this reported research work vouches for its application in the classification of AD.

Alzheimer's disease (AD) is reported as one of the primary cause of mental disabilities and ill-health worldwide. It is categorized into mild, moderate, and severe stages. Early detection and treatment of AD promises ample scope to control the rate of increase of neural disorders. The Structural Magnetic Resonance Imaging (MRI) is a diagnostic source for AD due to its high resolution and high contrast in depicting the brain's gray and white matter. Apart from this, physical and neurobiological examinations and observations in the form of Mini-Mental-State Examination (MMSE) and the patient's comprehensive record are also used for diagnosis and analysis.

7.2 ALZHEIMER'S DISEASE ANALYSIS USING ENSEMBLE CLASSIFIER (AD-EC)

The researchers have confirmed that the performance of classifiers can be improved using the principle of stacking. This research work aims to develop a single model, which is a composition of heterogeneous models.

This chapter explains the general framework for the analysis and prediction of Alzheimer's Disease (AD), based on a meta classifier using a logistic regression model.

They are three types of terms describing the ensemble models:

A. Bagging: To decrease the model's variance

B. Boosting: To decrease the model's bias.

C. Stacking: To increase the prediction force of the classifier

A. Bagging

The bagging model is used to decrease the variance and increase prediction accuracy. This model creates several subsets of data which is randomly selected from the training set.

B. Boosting

The boosting model is another ensemble technique that creates a group of predictions. The model learned sequentially through the early learner's fitting model. This model is used to analyze data and data errors. If the input data is irrelevant to the hypothesis, its weight is improved to attain better classification. Gradient boosting is an extension of the Gradient Descent over boosting method.

$$Gradient\ Boosting = Gradient\ Descent + Boosting$$

In this model, the gradient descent algorithm aims for minimum loss. The tree model's ensemble is built one by one, and the tree entities are included successively. If the tree tends to improve the loss, it signifies the dissimilarity between actual and predicted values. In this research work, a logistic regression model is used as a combinational scheme. Table 7.1 describes the comparison of Bagging, Boosting, and Stacking methods.

C. Stacking

Stacking is an ensemble learning technique that combines multiple classifications or regression models via a meta-classifier or a meta-regressor. The base-level models are trained based on a complete training set. Then the meta-model is trained on the outputs of the base level model-like features.

Table 7.1 Comparison of Bagging, Boosting, and Stacking

Feature	Bagging	Boosting	Stacking
Data from the subset	Randomly Selected	Misclassified samples gave higher preference	Diversified
Objective	Minimizes variance	Increases predictive force	Minimizes variance& Increases predictive force
Mechanics	Random subspace	Gradient descent	Blending
Model	(weighted) average	Weighted majority vote	Logistic regression

An outline of the basic functionalities of XGB, GBM, SVM, ETC, and KNN is given in the following section.

Extreme Gradient Boosting (XGB)

XGB utilizes several useful tricks, and it exceptionally handles structured data. The essential features are - computing and regularization. The computing method uses second-order gradients of the loss function. It obtains more information about the direction of gradients and obtains the minimum of the loss function. The base model - decision tree is an alternative for minimizing the error of the inclusive model. This model uses a second-order derivative as an estimator. The regularization (L1 & L2) is observed to get improved in this model. The additional advantages of the XG Boosting algorithm are fast training and parallelization across clusters. The three essential features of XGB are a model feature, system feature, and algorithm feature.

Model Features

Three primary gradient boosters support the model characteristics:

- The algorithm of Gradient boosting, also known as a Gradient boosting machine which includes the learning rate.
- Stochastic Gradient Boosts with row, column, and column sub-sampling at split levels.
- Regularized Gradient boosts with regularization in both L1 and L2.

System Feature:

The library offers a system which is used in a variety of computer environments, especially:

- Tree construction parallelization through the training of all CPU cores.
- The distributed computers with a machine cluster are essential for training complex models.
- Out –of- the-core computing for extensive memory-free datasets.
- Cache data structure optimization and algorithm to optimize hardware

Algorithm Features:

The algorithm is designed for calculation moment and memory resource effectiveness. A design objective was to make the best use of the resources available to train the model. Some main characteristics of the algorithm are:

- Automatically manage the missing information values with the sparse aware application.
- Structure block to promote tree building parallelization.
- Continued training to enhance a new information model already adapted.

Gradient Boosting Machine (GBM)

Two buzzwords, Bagging and Boosting, are frequently encountered while working with boosting algorithms. The term Bagging refers to the building of learning algorithms on random samples of data and taking simple means to determine bagging probabilities. On the other hand, the term Boosting refers to a similar process, but sample selection is carried out more intelligently, enabling us to increase the weights of hard-to-classify observations. The gradient booster classifier does boost as opposed to bagging. The observations are not chosen based on the bootstrap process but the errors. The prediction can be selected from among the models, such as decision trees, regressions, and classifiers. The new prediction learns from the inaccuracy produced by the previous predictors. It takes less time/iterations for real predictions. However, the stopping criteria should be chosen carefully, or the process could lead to overfitting on training data.

Support Vector Machine (SVM)

SVM is a supervised learning algorithm, suitable for both regression and classification. This algorithm anchors on the *hyper-plane* method. This method uses the minimum distance on the training data for classification. The data tends to have a liner hyper-plane between the two classes. The functions take low dimensional data input space and transform the same into a higher dimensional space. Therefore, the process of converting the data from non-separable to separable is cumbersome. These functions are called kernels and are used in non-linear separation problems.

Extra Trees Classifier (ETC)

Extra Trees Classifier is a decision tree model-based ensemble learning method, based on a. ETC model is more like a random forest method. It assumes certain decisions on subsets of data to minimize over-learning and overfitting.

Extra Trees is named for (Extremely Randomized Trees). Extra Trees Classifier adds another randomized step to the algorithm of the random forest.

Random forests calculate the ideal division into nodes using random feature subsets. For each feature within this random subset, a random division is enforced and, after comparing the randomly preferred divides, the best feature will subsequently be selected. These trees are f computationally complex than random forests and always performance comparable. The salient steps of this classifiers are given hereinunder.

1. Builds multiple trees with **bootstrap** = **False** by default, which means it samples without replacement.
2. Nodes are split based on **random** splits among a **random subset** of the features selected at every node.

K-Nearest Neighbours

The K-Nearest-Neighbour (KNN) classifier uses case-based learning for classification. It is an extension of the simple nearest neighbour technique. The main steps of K-Nearest-Neighbours implementation are:

(i) Similarity assessment: The performance comparison between the training and test set is calculated, either by the Euclidean distance, Manhattan distance, Jacquard similarity co-efficient, or correlation coefficient. Among these, the Euclidean distance method is mostly used for a given feature set ($x_{j1},x_{j2},\ldots,x_{ji}$) and training feature ($x_{j1},x_{j2},\ldots,x_{jn}$), the Euclidean distance is calculated as follows the Eqn.(7.1)

$$d_j = \sqrt{\sum_{i=1}^{n}(test_{ki} - train_{kn})} \tag{7.1}$$

where n is the number of feature vectors, k is the number of training and testing sample data. d_j is the Euclidean distance between the jth sample of the training and test data.

(ii) The vote and classification applied to the test sample dataset are classified based on every class's voting results.

Stacking Ensemble Learning

Binning, bagging, and stacking are the basic parts of a data scientist's toolkit and a part of a series of ML techniques, and so they are called ensemble methods.

Stacking is the combined progression of multiple classifiers generated by diverse learning algorithms $l_{1,} l_2, \dots \dots . l_n$ on a single dataset. A set of C1, C2.... Cn classifiers are produced during the first phase. A meta-level classifier to combine the base-level classifiers is implemented in the second phase.

Logistic Regression Model

The MLR (Multi response Linear Regression) algorithm has an advantage when used in stacking. This regression model is capable of handling categorical variables. It is used to estimate the probability results, based on the given features.

Logistic regression measures the relationship between the input variables and the results by estimating probabilities. The probability of Y given X is in Eqn. (7.2)

$$P(Y = 1|X = x) \qquad (7.2)$$

The meta classifier Logistic Regression is similar used to the linear regression. Then Eqn. (7.2) P for linear regression is given in Eqn. (7.3)

$$w_1x_1 + w_2x_2 + \cdots = \sum w_i x_i \qquad (7.3)$$

Logistic transformation is used to convert linear regression given by Eqn. (7.4) & Eqn. (7.5)

$$log \frac{P(x)}{1-P(x)} \qquad (7.4)$$

$$P = \frac{e^{\sum w_i x_i}}{1+e^{\sum w_i x_i}} = \frac{1}{1+e^{-\sum w_i x_i}} \qquad (7.5)$$

where 'p' is the logistic model predicted probability. The next step is to calculate the difference between these two log-likelihoods. Where w_i is the Wald's statistic with a normal distribution. Given some linear combination x_i of the predictors.

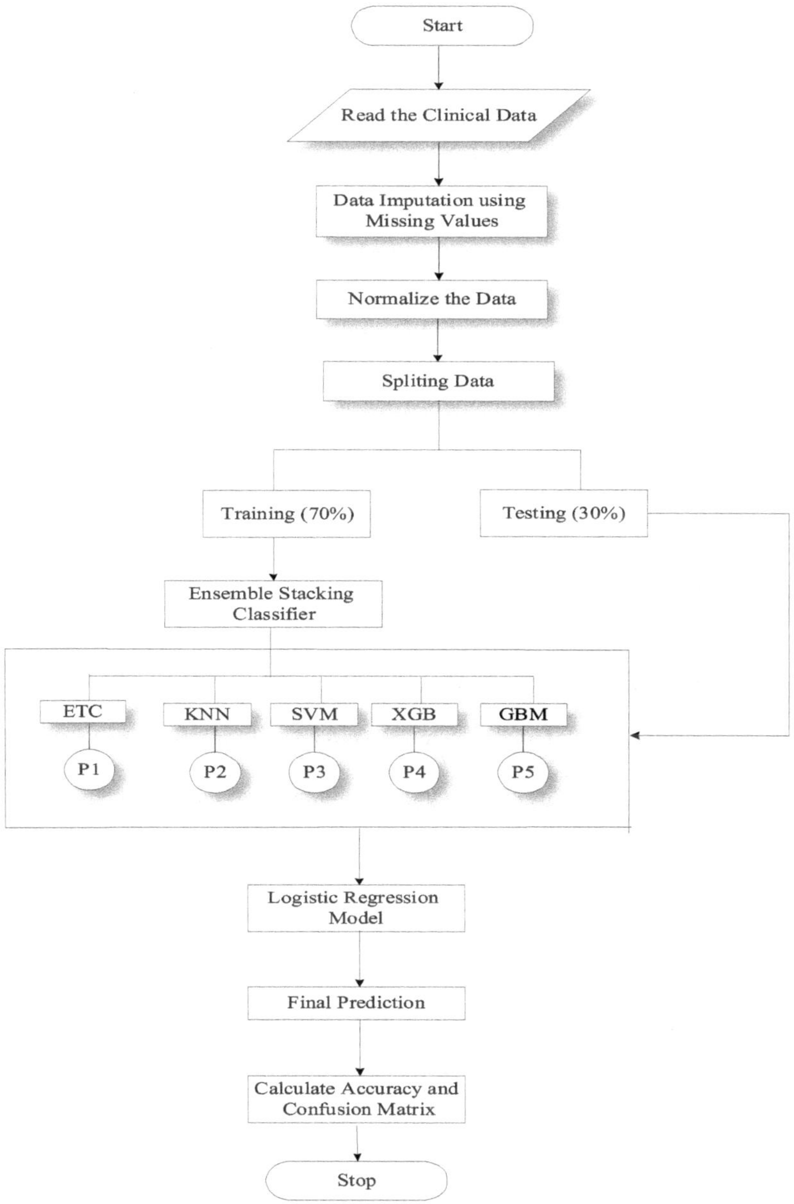

Fig. 7.1 Flow Diagram of the Proposed AD-EC

The flow diagram of AD-EC is given in Fig. 7.1 and its algorithmic description is given in Algorithm 7.1

7.1 Algorithmic Description for AD-EC

Input: Clinical Data

Output: Classification of AD stages

Phase – I: Pre-Processing

begin

Step 1: Read the clinical data

Step 2: Pre-Process using Data imputation for filling in missing values.

Step 3: One-Hot Encoding if categorical input data is found.

Step 4: Split data for training and testing.

Phase – II: Classification

Step 5: Train the dataset applies XGB, KNN, SVM, ETC, GBC classifier algorithms

Step 6: Apply Stacking algorithm

Step 7: Apply the logistic regression model and tune the hyperparameters

Step 8: Evaluate the performance of the proposed classifier algorithm using the test set.

end

7.2.1 RESULTS AND DISCUSSION

The classification report performance of Model 1, Model 2, Model 3, Model 4, and Model 5 in Tables 7.4, 7.5, 7.6, 7.7, and 7.8, respectively. The results declare that Model1, Model3, Model4, and Model5 models are top performers when compared with all other models. The ensemble of Model1,

Model3, Model4, and Model5 for our ultimate structural design. The ensemble model $Ensemble_1$ (Model1 + Model2), $Ensemble_2$ (Model3 + Model4+ Model5), $Ensemble_3$ (Model1 + Model2+ Model3+ Model 4) and $Ensemble_4$ (Model1 + Model2+ Model3+ Model4+ Model5) and the performance compared to the ensemble model of Model1, Model2, Model3, Model4, and Model5 are proposed.

The different classifiers were tested using the dataset described, and the classification precision, accuracy, Recall, F1-score were determined for each classifier. The results presented here will provide an evaluation for the execution of the dissimilar classifiers concerning each metric. The results obtained for each model are numerically recorded in Tables and respectively depicted as charts.

Table 7.2 Performance Analysis of Classification models

MODEL	SCORE (ACCURACY) %
Extra Tree Classifier (ETC) Model 1	0.80357 (80.35)
Support Vector Machine (SVM) Model 2	0.8125 (81.25)
K-Nearest Neighbour (KNN) Model 3	0.73214 (73.21)
Extreme Gradient Boosting (XGB) Model 4	0.82142 (82.14)
Gradient Boosting Machine (GBM) Model 5	0.83035 (83.03)

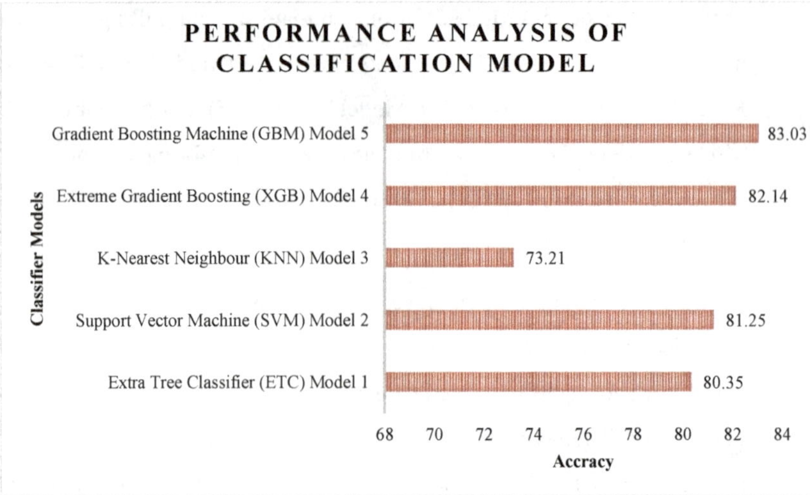

Fig. 7.2 Performance Analysis of Classifiers using Accuracy

Fig. 7.2 and Table 7.2 show a comparison of the classification accuracy obtained by various classifier models. It could be observed that KNN exhibits the lowest prediction levels, while GBT exhibits the highest prediction levels.

Case 1:

Table 7.3 shows the ensemble classifier $Ensemble_1$ models Precision, Recall, and F1-Score obtained by GBM and SVM classifier. The E_1 stacking classifier model's accuracy is 82.14%.

Table 7.3 Performance of Stacking Classifier $Ensemble_1$ (GBM & SVM)

Group	Precision	Recall	F1-Score	Support
Converted (0)	0.00	0.00	0.00	19
Demented (1)	0.82	1.00	0.90	40
Non-demented (2)	0.83	0.98	0.90	53
Classification model report				
Micro Avg.	0.82	0.82	0.82	112
Macro Avg.	0.55	0.66	0.60	112
Weighted Avg.	0.68	0.82	0.75	112
Accuracy: 0.821428 (82.14%)				

Case 2:

Table 7.4 shows the ensemble classifier $Ensemble_2$ models Precision, Recall, and F1-Score obtained by XGB, ETC, and KNN classifier. The E_2 stacking classifier model's accuracy is 83.05%.

Table 7.4 Performance of Stacking Classifier $Ensemble_2$ (XGB, ETC, & KNN)

Group	Precision	Recall	F1-Score	Support
Converted (0)	1.00	0.05	0.10	19
Demented (1)	0.83	1.00	0.91	40
Non-demented (2)	0.83	0.98	0.90	53
Classification model report				
Micro Avg.	0.83	0.83	0.83	112
Macro Avg.	0.89	0.68	0.64	112
Weighted Avg.	0.86	0.83	0.77	112
Accuracy: 0.83035(83.05%)				

Case 3:

Table 7.5 shows the ensemble classifier $Ensemble_3$ models Precision, Recall, and F1-Score obtained by XGB, ETC, KNN, and SVM classifier. The E_3 Stacking classifier model's accuracy is 82.14%. The accuracy decreased due to the usage of the SVM classifier.

Table 7.5 Performance of Stacking Classifier $Ensemble_3$ (XGB, ETC, KNN, & SVM)

Group	Precision	Recall	F1-Score	Support
Converted (0)	0.00	0.00	0.10	19
Demented (1)	0.82	1.00	0.90	40
Non-demented (2)	0.83	0.98	0.90	53
Classification model report				
Micro Avg.	0.82	0.82	0.82	112
Macro Avg.	0.55	0.66	0.60	112
Weighted Avg.	0.86	0.82	0.75	112
Accuracy: 0.821428 (82.14%)				

Case 4:

Table 7.6 shows the ensemble classifier $Ensemble_4$ models Precision, Recall, and F1-Score obtained by XGB, ETC, KNN, and GBM classifier. The E_4 stacking classifier model's accuracy is 91.07%.

Table 7.6 Stacking Classifier $Ensemble_4$ (XGB, ETC, KNN, & GBM)

Group	Precision	Recall	F1-Score	Support
Converted (0)	0.50	0.10	0.17	10
Demented (1)	0.90	1.00	0.95	46
Non-demented (2)	0.93	0.98	0.96	56
Classification Model Report				
Micro Avg.	0.91	0.91	0.91	112
Macro Avg.	0.78	0.69	0.69	112
Weighted Avg.	0.88	0.91	0.88	112
Accuracy: 0.91071 (91.07%)				

Case 5:

Table 7.7 shows the ensemble classifier Ensemble$_5$ models Precision, Recall, and F1-Score obtained by XGB, ETC, KNN, SVM, and GBM classifier. The proposed method with E_5 stacking classifier model accuracy is 92.85% to 93%.

Table 7.7 Stacking Classifier Ensemble$_5$ (XGB, ETC, KNN, SVM, & GBM)

Group	Precision	Recall	F1-Score	Support
Converted (0)	1.00	0.20	0.33	10
Demented (1)	0.92	1.00	0.96	46
Non-demented (2)	0.93	1.00	0.97	56
Classification Model report				
Micro Avg.	0.93	0.93	0.93	112
Macro Avg.	0.95	0.73	0.75	112
Weighted Avg.	0.93	0.93	0.91	112
Accuracy: 0.928571 (92.85%)				

The proposed method uses a Meta classifier, the logistic regression model, with hyperparameters tuning. The proposed model's accuracy is increased.

Fig. 7.3 and Table 7.8 shows the comparison of the classification models accuracy obtained by stacking ensemble classifiers. For a side-by-side comparison of the performance of the different classifiers, it uses five quality indicators. The analysis of every combination of modifier shows that the Ensemble 5 model exhibits high prediction levels, making it the best ensemble model for prediction.

Table 7.8 Performance Analysis of Ensemble Models using Accuracy

Ensemble Model	Accuracy (%)
Ensemble1(GBM and SVM)	82.14
Ensemble 2 (XGB, ETC, and KNN)	83.05
Ensemble 3 (XGB, ETC, KNN, and SVM)	82.41
Ensemble4(XGB, ETC, KNN, and GBM)	91.07
Ensemble5(XGB, ETC, KNN, SVM, and GBM)	92.85

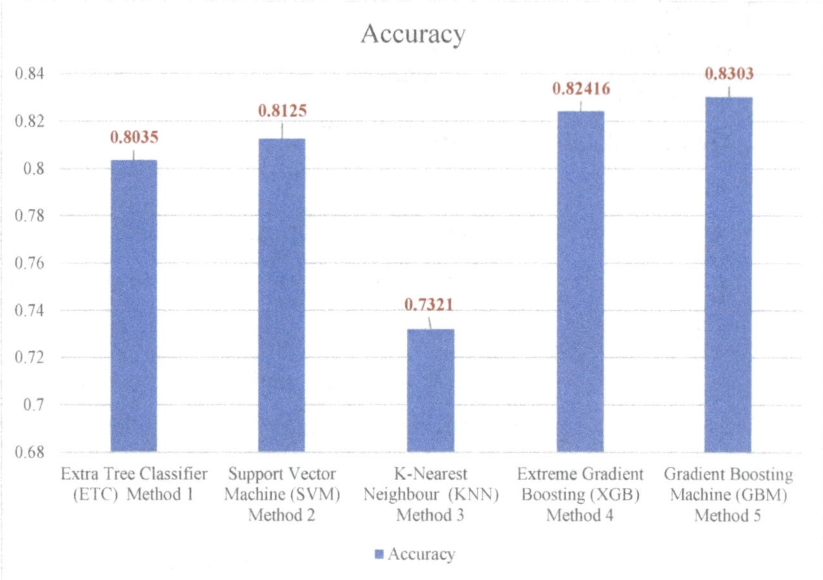

Fig. 7.3 Performance Analysis of Ensemble Models using Accuracy

For an overall comparison of the different classifiers' performance, six quality indicators defined are Scant, Poor, Low, Moderate, High, and Excellent. Each classifier exhibits a certain level of performance in a particular metric is discussed below.

T: Scant performance if value achieved is 0–9%;

Q: Poor performance if value achieved is 10–29%;

M: Low performance if value achieved is 30–49%;

N: Moderate performance if value achieved is 50–69%;

I: High performance if value achieved is 70–89%;

F: Excellent performance if value achieved is 90–100%

Table 7.9 Performance Summary of the Ensemble Stacking Classifiers

Metric / Classifier	Precision			Recall			F1-Score		
	C	D	ND	C	D	ND	C	D	ND
Ensemble $_1$	S	H	H	S	E	E	S	E	E
Ensemble $_2$	E	H	H	M	E	E	P	E	E
Ensemble $_3$	S	H	H	S	E	E	S	E	E
Ensemble $_4$	M	E	E	P	E	E	P	E	E
Ensemble $_5$	E	E	E	P	E	E	L	E	E

C: Converted; D: Demented; ND: Non-Demented

Excellent (E): 90-100; High (H): 70-89; Moderate (M): 50-69;

Low (L): 30-49; Poor (P) 10-29; Scant (S): 0-9

Table 7.9 summarizes this information for the five stacking classifiers in the three different metrics (Precision, Recall, and F1-Score) for the three classes (Converted, Demented, and Non-Demented). The ensemble classifiers perform at an excellent level for one metric for a particular class and do not perform well in the same metric for a different class. To visualize the above data for a side-by-side comparison of the classifiers. It assigns a quality index for the performance. It uses a 6-point scale, assigning values of 1 through 6 for the performance levels of Scant through Excellent. Fig. 7.4 compares the performance of the different ensemble classifiers when the metric used is Precision. An analysis of Precision indicates the E5 ensemble exhibits good Precision on all three classes, and hence it can provide highly effective results.

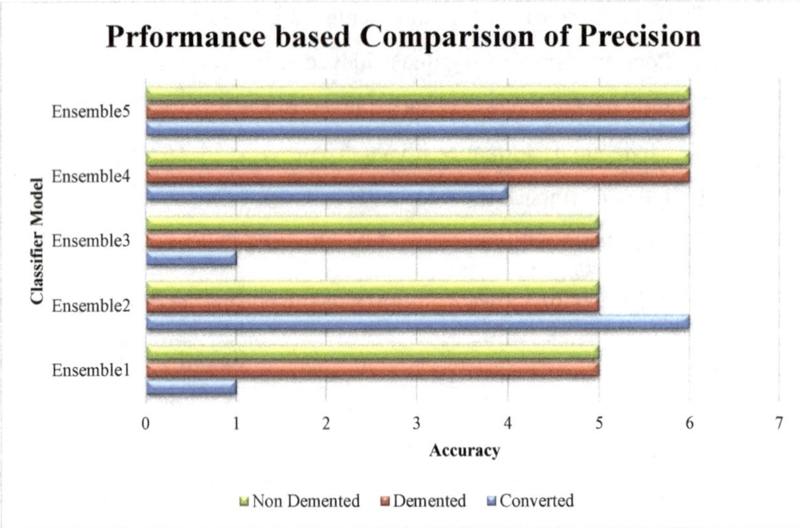

Fig. 7.4 Performance comparison based on Precision

Similarly, Fig. 7.5 compares the performance of the different classifiers based on Recall metrics. Although recall levels for the converted class are low, it is still higher than all the other models, making the Ensemble 5 classifier a good predictor even on complex classes.

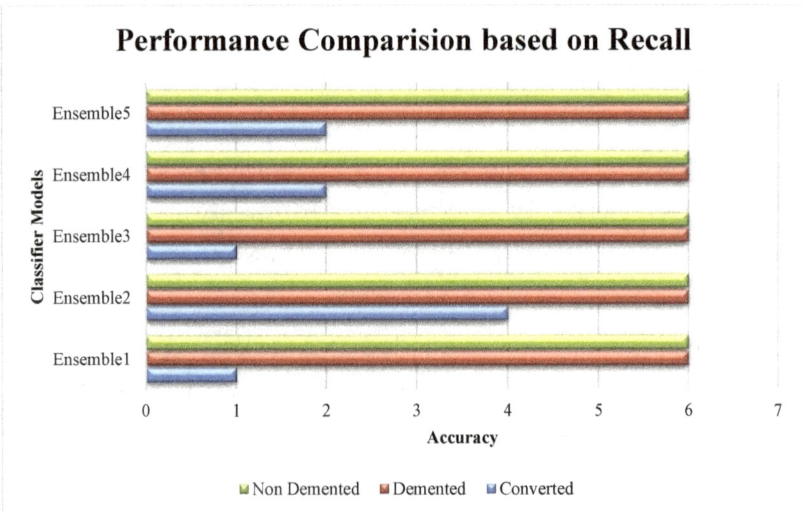

Fig. 7.5 Performance comparison based on Recall

Finally, Fig. 7.6 compares the performance of the different classifiers when using the F1-Score metric. F1 Score of the E5 model exhibits the best performance on all the classifier models, making it one of the best performers.

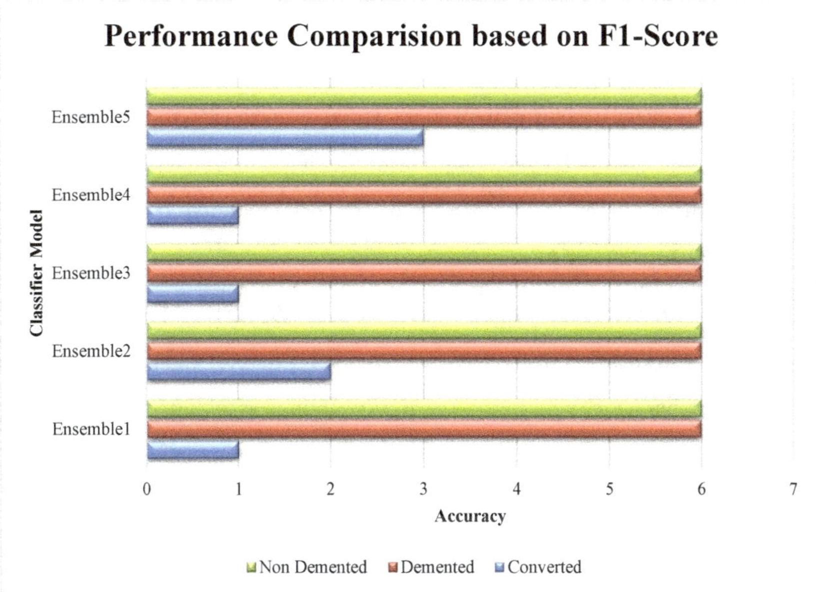

Fig. 7.6 Performance Comparison based on F1-Score

7.3 Alzheimer's Disease Detection using Random Forest Classifier with Hyper Parameters Tuning (AD-RFC-HPT)

In this chapter, a 4-way classifier, Healthy Control (HC), Mild Alzheimer's disease (AD), Very Mild AD, and Moderate AD persons are employed. Experiments are performed using the OASIS dataset, and the results are obtained for Multi-class classification of the disease. The performance of the random forest classifier model is confirmed to outperform its counterparts progressively. The improved accuracy of random forest classifiers experimented in this reported research work vouches for its application in the classification of the stages of AD.

7.3.1 METHODOLOGY OF AD-RFC-HPT

The Random Forest Classifier (RFC) performs regression tasks as well as classification tasks using a supervised learning approach. It undertakes dimensionality reduction and handles missing values, outliers, and other essential processes in data exploration. It may be considered a group learning method, where a group of weak models aggregates to form an efficient model.

Random Forest Hyperparameters: The hyperparameters in the random forest algorithm are used to accelerate the model's predictive power and increase the model's speed and effectiveness.

I. **Increasing the Predictive Power:** The hyperparameter n_estimators denotes the number of trees included in the algorithm before computing the majority voting or taking average values of the prediction labels. This algorithm's computation time is directly proportional to the number of trees, constituting the forest. While this approach helps to increase accuracy, it slows down the computation. The next hyperparameter, namely max _features, represents the maximum limit on the number of features allowed to try for Random Forest classification in an individual tree. The last hyperparameter, which is related to speed, is min _sample_leaf. The minimum amount of leaves needed to divide an inner node is shown in this parameter.

II. **Increasing the Model's Speed:** The n_jobs hyperparameter determines the number of processors used for parallel computation. When this parameter has a value of 1, it means only one processor can be used; a value of -1 means there is no limit on the number of processors. The hyperparameter random state determines the replicability of the output of the model. The model provides the same result on a definite value of random state and for the same hyperparameters and training data. The oob_score hyperparameter determines the cross-validation for the random forest model. In this cross-validation, one-third of the data is retained to test the model and not used for training. These retained samples are called out of the bag samples. The proposed RFC with hyperparameter tuning addresses overfitting and assures improved performance to change the value of bias and variance. This method of hyperparameter tuning has increased the predictive power of the model. The description of the hyperparameters and the permissible data values of each parameter are furnished

Hyperparameters Tuning used in the model

1. **n_estimators (data type: *integer*; data value: 5)**

   The number of trees in the forest.

2. **criterion: (data type: *string;* data value: 'Gini', 'Entropy')**

   The function measures the quality of a split. Supported criteria are "gini" for the Gini impurity and "entropy" for the information gain.

3. **max_depth : (data type: *integer;* data value: Min.: 5 & Max.:10)**

   The maximum depth of the tree. If None, then nodes are expanded until all leaves are pure or until all leaves contain less than min_samples_split samples.

4. **min_samples_split : (data type: *integer;* data value: 5)**

   The minimum number of samples required to split an internal node:

5. **min_samples_leaf : (data type: *integer;* data value: Min.: 7)**

   The minimum number of samples required to be at a leaf node. A split point at any depth will only be considered if there are at least min_samples_leaf training samples in each of the left and right branches. This may smoothen the model, especially in regression.

6. **max_leaf_nodes : (data type: *integer;* data value: Max.: 15)**

   Grow trees with max_leaf_nodes in best-first fashion. Best nodes are defined as relative reduction in impurity. Fig. 7.7 shows the flow of the proposed method.

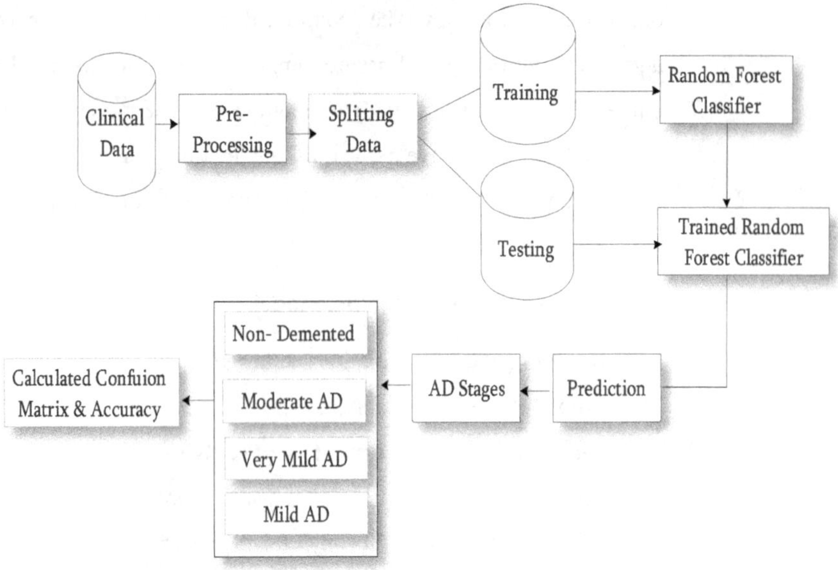

Fig. 7.7 Flowchart of AD-RFC-HPT

The flow diagram of AD-RFC-HPT is given in Fig.7.7 and its algorithmic description is given in algorithm 7.2

7.2 Algorithmic Description of AD-RFC-HPT

Input: Clinical Data

Output: Classification of AD stages

begin

Phase I: Pre-Processing

Step 1: Read the clinical data

Step 2: Clinical Data using Data Imputation using Pre-Processing Method

Step 3: Pre-Processing Data Apply Transformation

Step 4: Cleaning data using splitting for training and testing data

Phase II: Prediction

Step 5: Train and test the data using tuning hyperparameters random forest classifier algorithm

Step 6: Testing the predicted data in AD stages

Step 7: Calculated Confusion Matrix and Accuracy for model Performance

Step 8: Calculate Mean Absolute Error in Training and Testing Data for model performance

end

7.3.2 Results and Discussion

The Random Forest Classifier Algorithm was tested using the dataset described, and the Precision, Accuracy, Recall, and F1-score were determined for each classifier. The results presented here will provide an evaluation of the execution of the dissimilar classifier concerning each metric. The metrics are intended as the percentage of quality of correctly classified samples separated by the sum number of samples. The classification results have validated the effectiveness of AD-RFC-HPT.

Table 7.10 Performance Analysis of AD-RFC-HPT

Group	Precision	Recall	F1-Score	Support
Without Data Imputation				
Mild AD	0.29	0.33	0.31	12
Moderate AD	0.00	0.00	0.00	2
Non-Demented	0.52	0.61	0.56	59
Very Mild AD	0.34	0.24	0.29	41
With Data Imputation (Proposed)				
Mild AD	1.00	0.81	0.90	16
Moderate AD	0.00	0.00	0.00	2
Non-Demented	1.00	096	0.98	69
Very Mild AD	0.82	1.00	0.90	27
With Tuning Hyper Parameters (proposed)				
Mild AD	0.93	0.93	0.93	15
Moderate AD	0.00	0.00	0.00	1
Non-Demented	1.00	1.00	1.00	62
Very Mild AD	0.97	1.00	0.99	34
Classification Report				
Without Data Imputation (Accuracy: 44.64%)				
Micro Avg	0.38	0.40	0.39	112
Macro Avg	0.43	0.45	0.43	112
With Data Imputation (Accuracy: 94.64%)				
Micro Avg	0.94	0.92	0.92	112
Macro Avg	0.96	0.95	0.95	112
With Tuning Hyper Parameter (Accuracy: 98.21%)				
Micro Avg	0.73	0.73	0.73	112
Macro Avg	0.97	0.98	0.98	112

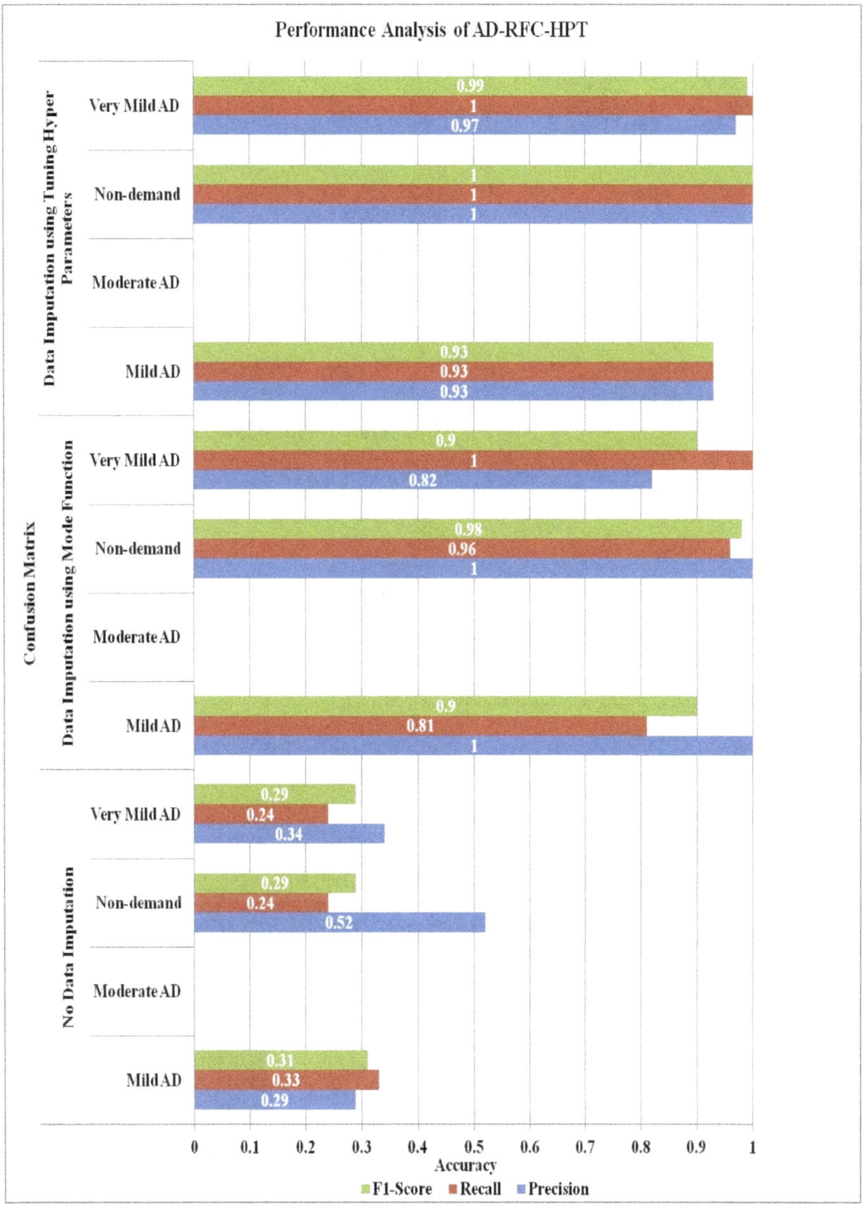

Fig. 7.8 Performance Analysis of AD-RFC-HPT

Performance analysis of the proposed method AD-RFC-HPT is shown in Fig. 7.8 and Table 7.10.

In No-Data Imputation, predictions were found to be low, and the accuracy level was also observed to be very low. Data Imputation can be observed to exhibit a positive impact on the model of data imputation using mode function. In this model, the accuracy level increase of 50% is observed.

The accuracy is shown an increase of 4%, and the other performance metrics also show improved performance exhibiting the efficiency of the data imputation using Tuning Hyper Parameters.

Table 7.11 Performance Analysis of Support

	Mild AD	**Moderate AD**	**Non-Demented**	**Very Mild AD**
Without Data Imputation	12	2	59	41
With Data Imputation	16	2	69	27
With Hyper Parameters Tuning	15	1	62	34

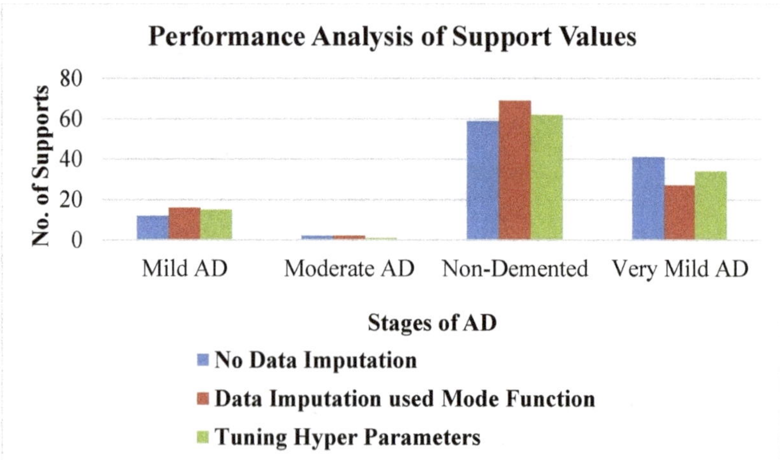

Fig. 7.9 Performance Analysis of Support Values

The supports are a quantitative metric that counts on the number of images considered by RFC during classification against the total No. of image count in experimented data. These results are visually being annotated in Table 7.11 and Fig. 7.9. The micro average denotes the accuracy of true positive (Precision), and the macro average is a measure of accuracy on false positive (Recall). In the OASIS dataset with 448 data, 112 data are of Mild AD, 112 data are Moderate AD, 112 data are Non-Demented and 112 data are Very Mild AD-affected ones. The AD-RFC-HPT model is accurately supported by all the data in the clinical dataset, as depicted by the observed support values.

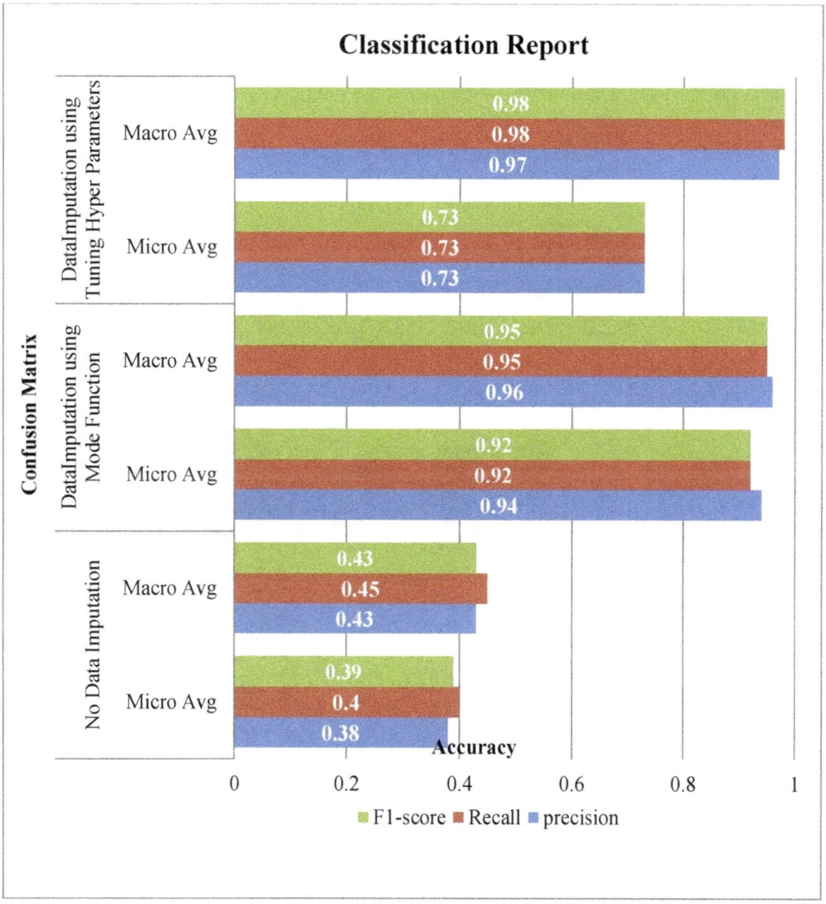

Fig. 7.10 Classification Analysis of AD-RFC-HPT

Table 7.12 Performance analysis of RFC Models

Model	Accuracy
RFC	95%
RFC-HPT	98%

Classification Analysis of AD-RFC-HPT is shown in Fig. 7.10. Fig. 7.11 and Table 7.12 show a comparison of the classification model accuracy obtained by the RFC and AD-RFC-HPT classifier. It could be observed that the RFC-HPT provides excellent performance compared to the RFC model.

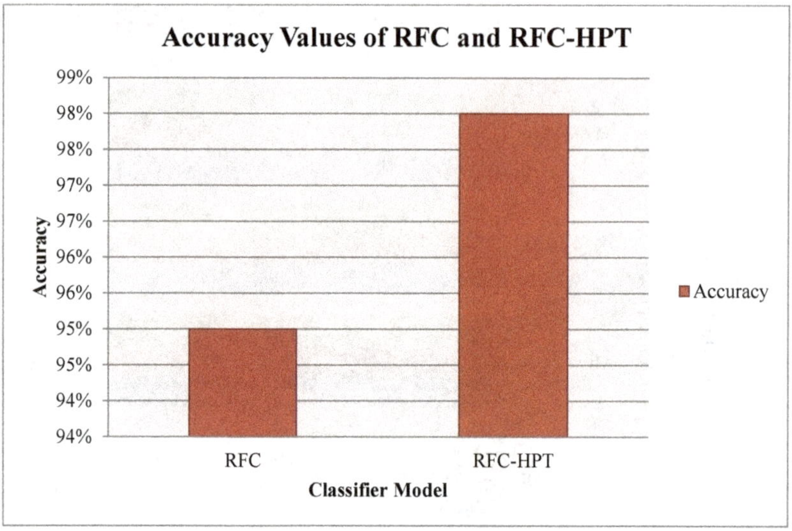

Fig. 7.11 Performance Analysis of RFC and RFC- HPT based on Accuracy

7.4 CONCLUSION

This research work reports the improved efficiency of the ensemble model using five techniques: Extra Tree Classifier (ETC), K-Nearest-Neighbor Classifier (KNN), Support Vector Machine (SVM), Extreme Gradient Boosting (XGB), and Gradient Boosting Machine (GBM). This multi-class classification approach is proved to promise higher accuracy than their classification models. The models are tested on the Normal and AD dataset. The accuracy of the ensemble assures Precision on early-stage AD diagnosis.

From this perspective of classification techniques, two primary components are divisible: preprocessing and classification. The pre-processing includes the data imputation method using the statistical mode function. The classification is done using Random Forest Classifier with Hyperparameters Tuning (AD-RFC-HPT) algorithms for AD's early diagnosis stages.

CHAPTER 8

OPTIMIZED CONVOLUTIONAL NEURAL NETWORK FOR ALZHEIMER'S DISEASE CLASSIFICATION

8.1 INTRODUCTION

Convolution Neural Network (CNN) is of deep learning technique that plays a vital role in image processing applications such as object identification, recognition, detection, and classification. Deep Learning techniques are capable of learning feature representations from the data. A CNN model takes images as the input, applies convolution operation(s), and extracts the image features, resulting in dimensionality reduction of the input. Those extracted features directly influence the accuracy of image processing.

Early detection and accurate analysis of Alzheimer's disease paves the way for strategic decisions on suitable therapeutic procedures. This chapter describes the optimization of a CNN model, with hyperparameter fine-tuning, to improve the degree of accuracy and minimize the error rate in AD detection. The CNN model is designed as a binary classifier that classifies the images into Healthy Control (HC) and AD.

AD is a type of dementia and the primary cause of physical and mental disability. This chapter considers the three most essential patterns of Alzheimer's disease: mild, moderate, and severe [NIH USA (2013)]. The early detection of AD is needed to provide on-time treatment for the patients.

MR brain images provide intrinsic details about the brain and exhibit high-resolution and high contrast on gray matter, the white matter of the brain, cerebrospinal fluid, and other brain anatomical structures. Hence, the experimental model was tested on the MIRIAD dataset, and the obtained results are recorded to ascertain its merits. The performance is evaluated using metrics, namely Accuracy, Precision, Recall, and F1-Score.

8.2 METHODOLOGY OF AD-OCNN

Convolution Neural Network is used to implement a deep learning framework [Wen, J 2019]. It consists of discrete elements called neurons, which are interconnected and arranged as layers. The Neural Network (NN) is a machine learning algorithm built on the concept of logistics and biological neural network functions.

The basic neural network architecture is shown in Fig. 8.1.

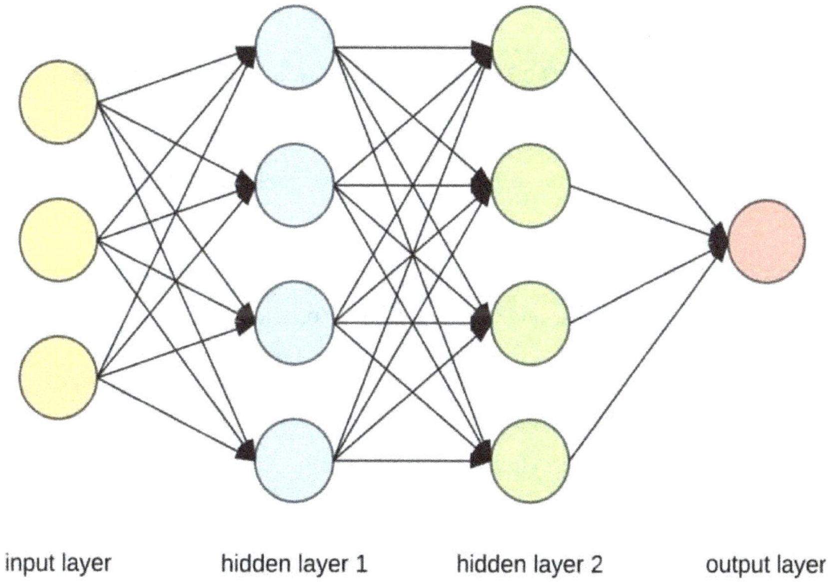

Fig. 8.1 Basic Neural Network Architecture

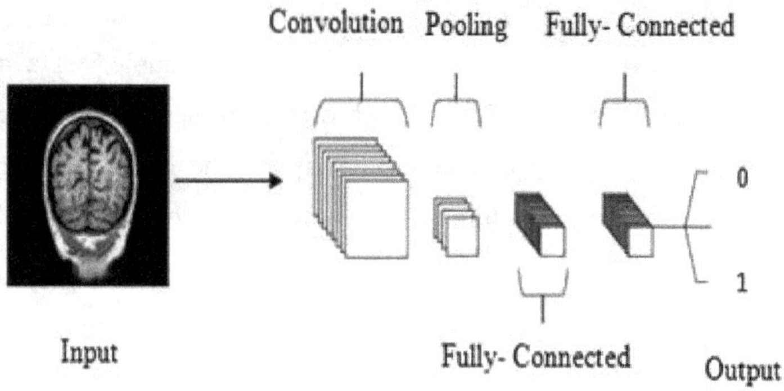

Fig. 8.2 Image Classification using the CNN model

CNN is a special architecture of Artificial Neural Network which is used to characterize the visual cortex. It is the most accepted architecture for image classification is shown in Fig.8.2. The CNN uses the following layers: Convolutional layer, non-linear, pooling layer, dropout layer, flatten and fully connected layers, and the output layer produced to detect the AD [Basaia, S 2019].

1. **Convolutional layers:** Convolution layer is used to extract the characters from the input image [Sambath Kumar S. 2017]. The convolutional layer maintains the association connects pixels by learning image features from input data. The mathematical operation takes two input image matrices and a 3×3 kernel filter. The 5×5 image pixel values and the convolution filter of 3×3 are given in Fig. 8.3.

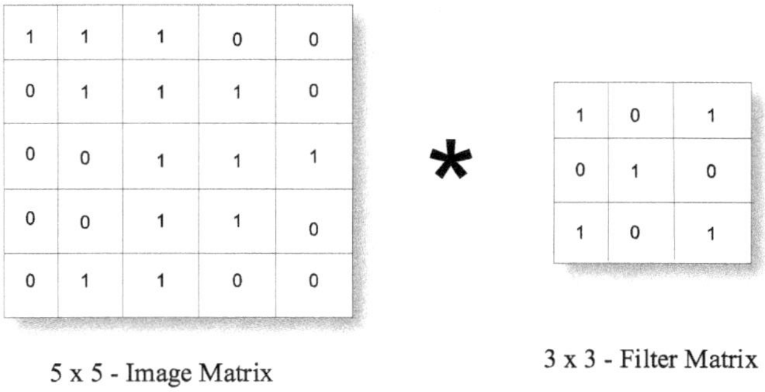

Fig. 8.3 Illustration of Image Convolution (a) Input Image (b) Convolution Mask

2. **Nonlinear Layer (ReLU):** The ReLU stands for Rectified Linear Unit for a non-linear operation. The ReLU is given in Eqn. (8.1)

   $f(x) = max(0, x)$ (8.1)

   The ReLU's purpose is to introduce non-linearity in the CNN. The CNN allows learning non-negative linear values, using the ReLU function. Data scientists find that ReLU is better than the other two functions, such as tanh, sigmoid. Fig. 8.4 shows the operation of ReLU.

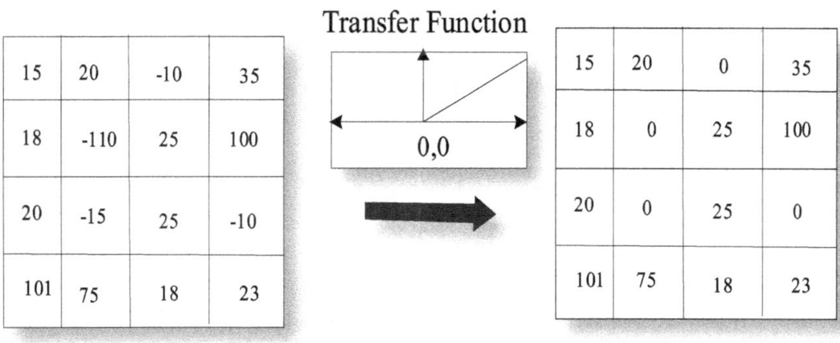

Fig. 8.4 ReLU Operation

3. **Pooling Layer:** The pooling layer reduces the spatial size, reducing the parameters and computational load. The spatial pooling is also called subsampling and down sampling. The spatial pooling can be of different types:
   (i) Max-Pooling
   (ii) Average-Pooling
   (iii) Sum-Pooling

   The proposed CNN method uses Max-Pooling, which takes the largest element from the rectified feature map, and it is shown in Fig. 8.5.

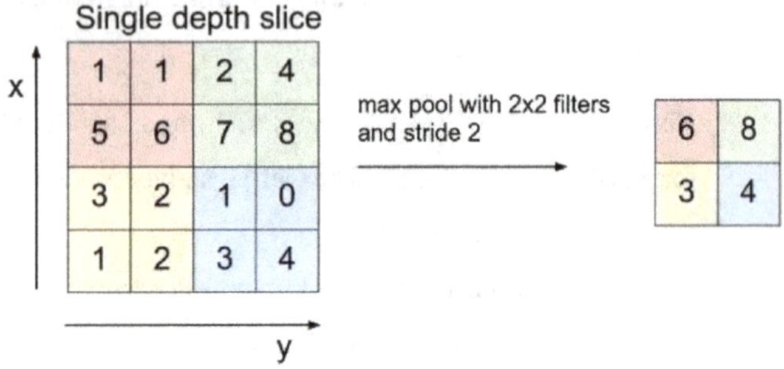

Fig. 8.5 Illustration of Max-Pooling Layer

4. **Dropout layer:** The dropout layer is used to avoid overfitting in the CNN model. The proposed model takes the dropout as 0.8.
5. **Fully-Connected Layer:** The final output layer is typically a fully connected neural network layer; the convolutional layer, ReLU, and Max-pooling layers are repeated as per the architecture of the CNN.

Fig.8.6, Fig.8.7, and Fig.8.8 depict the workflow, architecture, and schematic description of the CNN models. The proposed optimal Convolutional Neural Network is added to the fully connected layer with the non-linear sigmoid function.

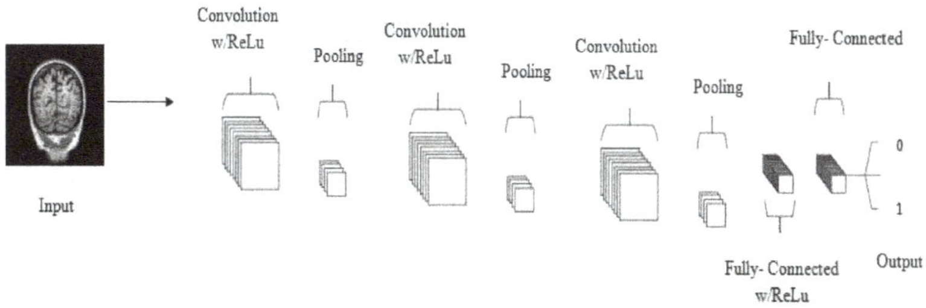

Fig .8.6 Proposed Optimal Convolutional Neural Network

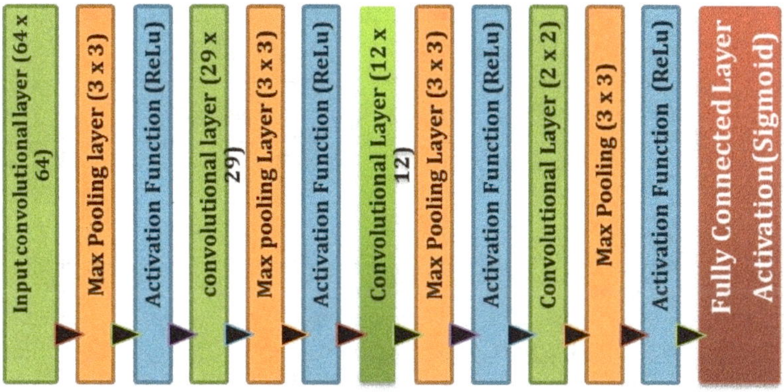

Fig. 8.7 Architecture of Proposed CNN Model

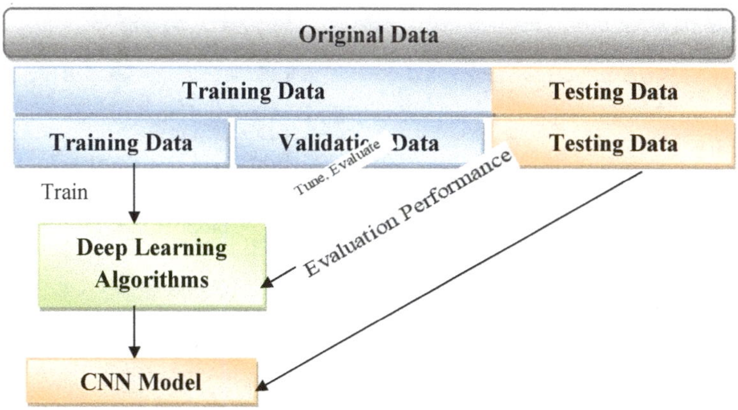

Fig. 8.8 Optimized CNN Model (proposed)

The details of the layers of CNN, convolution functions, activation, functions, and other functional components are listed in Table 8.1.

Table 8.1 Summary of CNN Model

Layer Type	Output_shape	Param #
Conv2d_1(conv2D)	(None, 256,256,32)	1568
Activation_1(Activation)	(None, 256,256,32)	0
Max_pooling2d_1 (Max Pooling 2)	(None, 256,256,32)	0
Dropout_1 (dropout 2)	(None, 256,256,32)	0
Conv2d_2(conv2D)	(None, 256,256,32)	32832
Activation_2(Activation)	(None, 256,256,32)	0
Max_pooling2d_2 (Max Pooling 2)	(None, 256,256,32)	0
Dropout_2(dropout 2)	(None, 256,256,32)	0
Conv2d_3(conv2D)	(None, 256,256,32)	233200
Activation_3(Activation)	(None, 256,256,32)	0
Max_pooling2d_3 (Max Pooling 2)	(None, 256,256,32)	0
Dropout_3(dropout 2)	(None, 256,256,32)	0
Conv2d_4(conv2D)	(None, 256,256,32)	524566
Activation_4(Activation)	(None, 256,256,32)	0
Max_pooling2d_4 (MaxPooling 2)	(None, 256,256,32)	0
Dropout_4(dropout 2)	(None, 256,256,32)	0
Flatten_1 (flatten)	(None, 200)	8663000
Dense_1(dense)	(None, 200)	0
Activation_5(Activation)	(None, 200)	0
Dropout_5(Dropout)	(None, 3)	201
Activation_6(Activation)	(None,3)	0

8.2.1 RESULTS AND DISCUSSION

Table 8.2 Performance Measures of CNN Models.

Group	Precision	Recall	F1-Score	Support
CNN Model				
Normal (0)	0.00	0.30	0.47	102
AD (1)	0.59	1.00	0.74	102
4-Layer CNN (Proposed)				
Normal (0)	0.87	0.73	0.79	102
AD (1)	0.76	0.89	0.82	102
.5-Layer CNN (Proposed)				
Normal (0)	1.00	0.21	0.34	102
AD (1)	0.56	1.00	0.72	102
Classification Report				
CNN Model (Accuracy: 0.65)				
Micro Avg	0.65	0.65	0.65	204
Macro Avg	0.79	0.65	0.60	204
Weighted Avg	0.79	0.65	0.60	204
4-Layer CNN Model (Accuracy: 0. 81)				
Micro Avg	0.81	0.81	0.81	204
Macro Avg	0.82	0.81	0.81	204
Weighted Avg	0.82	0.81	0.81	204
5-Layer CNN Model (Accuracy: 0. 60)				
Micro Avg	0.60	0.60	0.60	204
Macro Avg	0.78	0.60	0.53	204
Weighted Avg	0.78	0.60	0.53	204

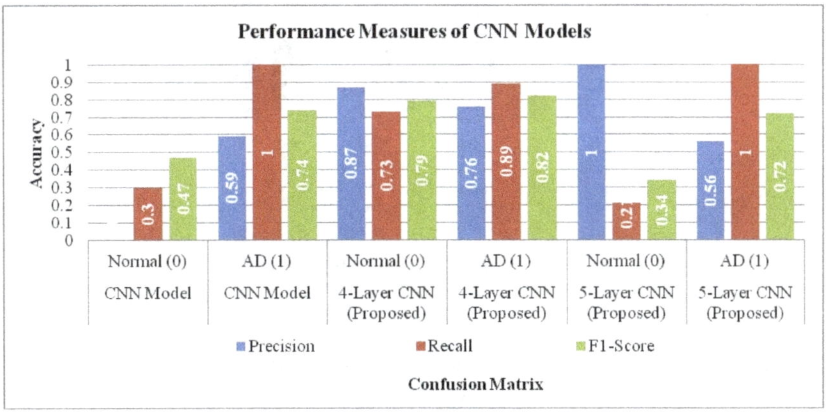

Fig. 8.9 Performance Measures of CNN Models

Table 8.2 and Fig. 8.9 show that a progressive increase in the layers has resulted in overtraining, where the normal class gets predicted accurately, whereas the AD class exhibits low performance.

The AD detection accuracy of the CNN model is 65%. The proposed optimized model with 4-layer has assured 80.88%, and CNN with five layers is 60.29%. These observations indicate that the proposed 4-layer CNN has exhibited an increased accuracy of 21%. This analysis proves that the four layer-CNN model is the best architecture for AD detection. These results are visually being annotated in Fig. 8.10 and 8.11. The micro average denotes the accuracy of true positive (Precision), the macro average is a measure of accuracy on false positive (Recall), and the weighted average is a measure of F1-Score. The support is a quantitative metric that counts on the number of images considered by CNN during classification against the total number of image count in the experimental dataset. In the MIRIAD dataset with 204 images, 102 images are normal, and 102 are AD-affected ones. The CNN model is accurately supported by all the dataset images, as depicted by the observed support values.

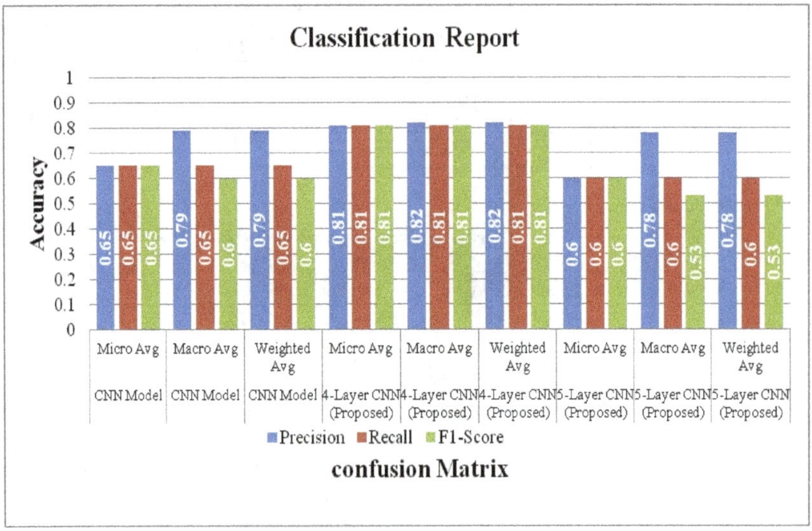

Fig. 8.10 Performance Analysis of Classification

Fig. 8.10 shows the classification report of the CNN layer.

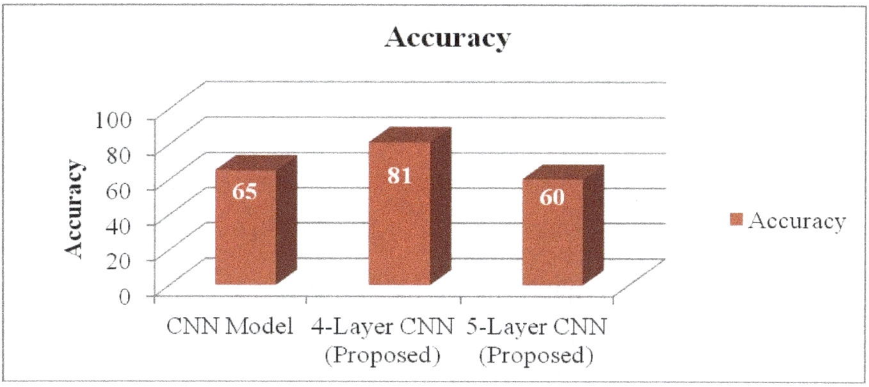

Fig. 8.11 Performance Analysis of Accuracy

8. 3 OPTIMIZED TRANSFER LEARNING (OTL)

This section describes the proposed optimized transfer learning (OTL) model on VGG16 for AD classification.

CNN gains attention for robust feature extraction and information mining. For a variety of applications such as object recognition, image super-resolution, and semantic segmentation. The Alex Net, VGG16, and VGG19 are the famous CNN architectures introduced for the object recognition task. In this chapter, the transfer learning is used to fine-tune the pre-trained network (VGG16) parameters for the image classification task. Performance evaluation was carried out using average recall, precision, and F-score. Performance analysis shows that fine-tuned VGG16 architecture outperforms the other CNN and hybrid learning approaches for the image classification task.

8.3.1 Methodology of OTL

Transfer learning is another machine learning principle where a model developed for a task is reused as the starting point for a model on a second task. It is a popular approach in deep learning where pre-trained models are used as the starting point on computer vision and natural language processing tasks. The two common approaches of Deep learning are:

- Develop a Model Approach

- Pre-trained Model Approach

Develop a Model Approach

Select Source Task. A related predictive modeling problem should be selected with an abundance of data where there is some relationship in the input data, output data, and concepts learned during the mapping from input to output data.

Develop Source Model. Next, A skillful model should be developed for the first task. The model must be better than a naive model to ensure that some feature learning has been performed.

Reuse Model. The model fit on the source task can then be used as the starting point for a model on the second task of interest. This approach may involve using all or parts of the model, depending on the mechanics of the modeling.

Tune Model. Optionally, the model may need to be adapted or refined on the input-output pair data available for the task of interest.

Pre-trained Model Approach

Select the Source Model. A pre-trained source model is chosen from available models. Many research institutions release models for large and challenging datasets and are added to the pool of candidate models.

Reuse Model. The pre-trained model can then be used as the starting point for a model on the second task of interest. This mechanism may involve using all or parts of the model, depending on the modeling technique used.

Tune Model. Optionally, the model is adapted or fine-tuned on the input-output pair data available for interest.

8.12 shows the optimal transfer learning architecture. The model was validated with OASIS. The classification technique chosen was SVM.

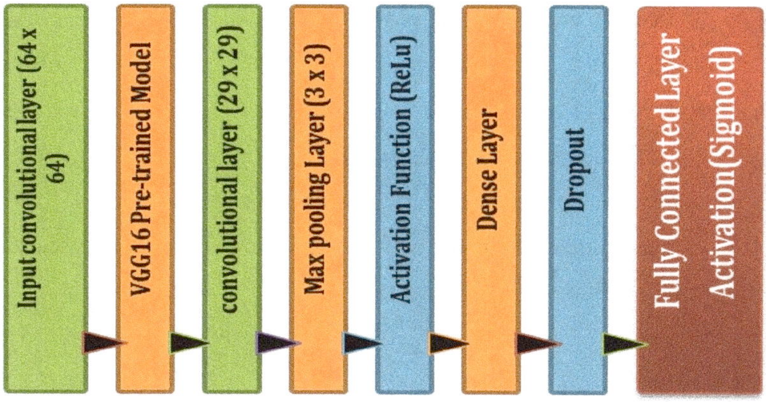

Fig. 8.12 Proposed Architecture OTL-VGG16

Table 8.3 Performance Measure of OTL

Group	**Precision**	**Recall**	**F1-Score**	**Support**
VGG16				
Normal (0)	1.00	0.52	0.68	162
AD (1)	0.24	1.00	0.38	24
OTL (Proposed)				
Normal (0)	0.93	0.91	0.97	102
AD (1)	0.92	0.89	0.95	102
Classification Report				
VGG16 Model (Accuracy: 0.58)				
Micro Avg	0.62	0.76	0.53	186
Macro Avg	0.96	0.58	0.64	186
OTL (Accuracy: 0. 91)				
Micro Avg	0.90	0.91	0.91	204
Macro Avg	0.92	0.91	0.91	204

The results obtained for VGG16 are listed in Table 8.3, and the respective plot is given Fig. 8.13. shows that an increase in the number of layers has resulted in overtraining, though the normal class gets predicted accurately. The accuracy of VGG16 model is 58%. The accuracy of the VGG16 model with five dense layers is 91%. Improved performance could be observed in both classes on the prediction of AD class. The recorded values endorse that the classification of both classes, namely Normal and AD are very good. Further, the higher values of micro and macro average recorded in the experimental study confirm that the proposed optimized model performs classification with increased accuracy.

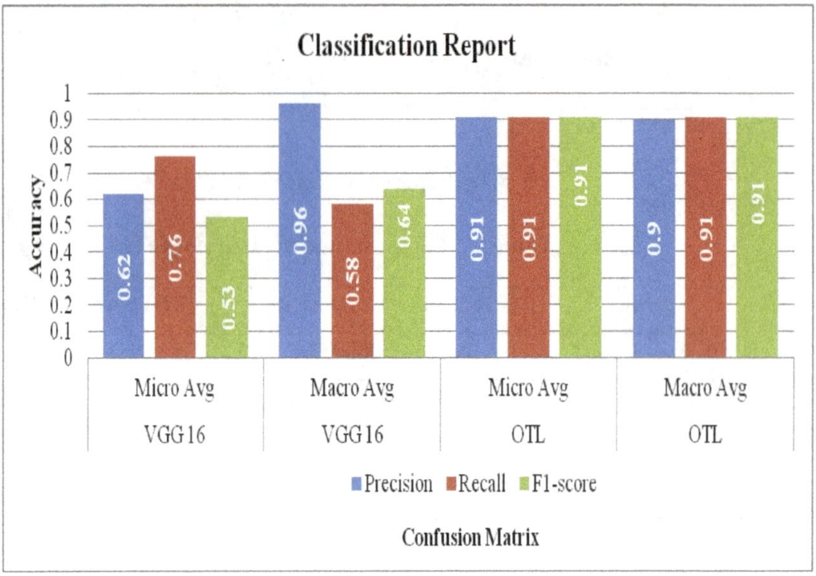

Fig. 8.13 Performance Analysis of Transfer Learning Model on VGG16

The results obtained for the OTL model is shown in Table 8.3 and Fig. 8.13. An improved performance depicted by the proposed model vouches for very high improvement in the prediction of AD class could be observed from the results. The recorded values endorse the fact performance level is both classes, namely Normal and AD are very good. Moreover, the higher values of micro and macro average confirm on the augmented performance of classification.

8.4 CONCLUSION

From the observation, it is evident that OTL classification on VGG16 produces an accuracy of 91.43, which is higher that of 4-layer CNN with 81% accuracy. Likewise, the respective results of Precision, Recall, F1-Score, Support, Micro-average, Macro-average, Weighted-average, and Overall-average endorse the fact that the optimized 4-Laye CNN and OTL-VGG16 have shown an appreciable increase in the accuracy of classification. Further, this experimental research observations highlight that subjective augmentation of layers may result in overfitting. The principle of transfer learning has substantially impacted the accuracy of classification.

CHAPTER 9

SUMMARY OF CONCLUSIONS

Alzheimer's Disease (AD) is one of the major causes of mortality among aged men and women in developed and developing countries. Early detection of AD provides enormous scope to reduce the death toll. MR brain images' clinical and research prospects have opened-up enormous avenues to design and develop new algorithms for segmentation, classification, and analysis of MR brain images. The research's objective is to develop new methods for early detection and diagnosis of AD from clinical and medical image datasets. Additionally, noise suppression for MR brain images also poses challenges of developing objective noise suppression techniques.

Every Computer-Assisted Diagnostic (CAD) system requires high performance and precise computational solutions for pre-processing the MR images for noise suppression and MR brain image segmentation and AD detection. The automated monitoring system for MRI brain image analysis demands the development of novel mechanisms for change detection between the various AD stages.

This thesis's research framework includes the development of ten computational procedures, under the broad spectrum of five different operations:

A. Noise Suppression

- Progressive Median Switching Filter (PMSF)

B. MR Brain Image Segmentation

- Thresholded and Morphological Operations Based Brain Image Segmentation (TMOS)
- MR Brain image segmentation using k-Means clustering and Expectation Maximization (MRB-kM-EM).

C. Alzheimer's Disease Detection from Clinical Datasets

- Alzheimer's Disease Classification using Multinomial Logistic Regression Classifier (AD-MNLR)

- Alzheimer's Disease Classification using Gradient Boosting Classifier with Hyper Parameters Tuning (AD-GBC-HPT)
- Alzheimer's Disease Classification using Decision Tree Classifier with Hyper Parameters Tuning (AD-DTC-HPT)
- Alzheimer's Disease Classification using Ensemble Classifier with Hyper Parameters Tuning (AD-EC-HPT)
- Alzheimer's Disease Classification using Random Forest Classifier with Hyper Parameters Tuning (AD-RFC-HPT)

D. Optimized Alzheimer's Disease Classification

- Optimized Convolutional Neural Network Model (AD-CNN)
- Optimized Transfer Learning Model (AD-OTL)

The proposed noise reduction and segmentation algorithms were developed using Matlab. The machine learning models were implemented using Python. The performance of segmentation was ascertained using Jaccard and Dice. The classification performance was ascertained using Precision, Recall and F1-Score, Support, Micro- average, Macro-average, Weighted-average, and Accuracy.

The datasets used for the experimental study are OASIS, MIRIAD, and IBSR.

This research's salient contributions are the fine-tuned and optimized intelligent machine learning models for feature extraction from the AD dataset/ image dataset and classification of AD into Mild AD; Moderate AD; and Non-Demented.

. The preprocessing operations, namely noise suppression, removal artifacts, and data imputation were performed suitably on clinical datasets and image datasets.

The skull stripping by TMOS has exhibited promising results that are endorsed by human visual perception.

The results of MRB-kM-EM exhibit its merit on brain image segmentation into the gray and white matter as measured by Jaccard and Dice. The Accuracy of similarity is obtained at 91% and 87% for Jaccard and Dice, respectively.

The machine learning classifier models, namely decision tree classifier, random forest classifier, gradient boosting classifier, ensemble classifier, and multinominal logistic regression, were experimented with hyperparameter tuning. The CNN and VGG16 classifier models were also optimized to improve the performance.

The seven AD classification techniques, namely Multinomial Logistic Regression with Hyper Parameters Tuning (AD-MNLR-HPT), Gradient Boosting Classifier with Hyper Parameters Tuning (AD-GBC-HPT), Decision Tree Classifier with Hyper Parameters Tuning (AD-DTC-HPT), Ensemble Classifier with Hyper Parameters Tuning (AD-EC-HPT), Random Forest Classifier with Hyper Parameters Tuning (AD-RFC-HPT), Optimized Convolutional Neural Network (AD-OCNN) and Optimized Transfer Learning (AD-OTL) are designed and developed under this research. Among them, the DTC-HPT gave the best results with the Accuracy of 99.10%, and RFC-HPT has produced 98.21% of Accuracy.

Further, the experimental results of Ensemble classifier AD-EC-HPT have assured the Accuracy of 92.85%.

The Accuracy of classification by GBC-HPT was 96%, which is yet another promising research outcome of this research.

The CNN model-based classification was evaluated in three flavors as the basic model; 4-layer CNN; and 5-Layer CNN. Those models produced the 65.89, 80.88%, and 60.29% of Accuracy, respectively. The 4-layer CNN has given the highest Accuracy. Moreover, it is observed that the 5-Layer model suffers from the additional overhead of overfitting.

The experimental results of transfer learning with VGG16 has depicted that the Accuracy of classification was 91.43%, whereas VGG16 could produce 58.01%.

This research work has substantially contributed to the development of high performing computational solutions using traditional and machine learning methods.

The improved Accuracy obtained for segmentation and classification in the process of AD detection is a valuable contribution to the automatic detection of Alzheimer's Disease. As the best experimental results obtained are 95% and above, the respective methods assure importance in AD detection and classification. Hence, incorporation of these smart algorithms in the AD detection trials will assist the radiologist and medical practitioners on AD detection.

Future Scope of the Research Work

Despite the merits of the proposed algorithms, such as computational simplicity and Accuracy of AD diagnosis and classification, this research domain has prospective opportunities for furthering the work. The proposed method's potentials can be augmented to handle complex and voluminous datasets and multi-class for AD detection with the bifold objectives of maximizing the accuracy of diagnosis and classification and minimizing the error rate.

CPSIA information can be obtained
at www.ICGtesting.com
Printed in the USA
LVHW080102060123
736479LV00006B/731